Need to Know Basics—
Dieting

Christopher D. Hudson

Katie E. Gieser

Christine Collier Erickson

Tim Baker

Carol Smith

Camille L. Steiner, MS FNP

Kristin Hillinger

BARBOUR
PUBLISHING

ISBN 1-58660-994-7

Check out Barbour's exciting web site at www.barbourbooks.com

Produced with the assistance of the Livingstone Corporation (www.Livingstonecorp.com). Project staff includes Joel Bartlett, Christopher D. Hudson, Kirk Luttrell, Ashley Taylor, and Rosalie Krusemark.

Interior Design by Design Corps, Batavia, IL.

Cover Design by Robyn Martins.

Cover and Interior Artwork by Elwood Smith.

Published by Barbour Publishing, Inc., P.O. Box 719, Uhrichsville, OH 44683

Our mission is to publish and distribute inspirational products offering exceptional value and biblical encouragement to the masses.

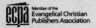 Member of the Evangelical Christian Publishers Association

Printed in the United States of America.
5 4 3 2 1

Table of Contents

Introduction vii

Section 1
Warm Welcome to All Dieters 1

Cliff Divers Wanted.....3
Welcome, Newbies!.....4
A Rockin' Appearance.....6
What Do You Want?.....9
Ranking Priorities.....12
Recognizing Weaknesses.....14
Setting Realistic Goals and Time Frames.....15

Section 2
What to Expect 17

Overview of the Book.....19

Section 3
Nutrition 23

The Classic Food Pyramid.....25
Pyramid Contents.....26
Count Your Servings.....28
Don't Forget Your Fruits and Veggies!.....29
Eat Your Veggies!.....30
Feeling Fruity?.....31
Health Issues.....32
Different Choices.....33
Diet Quiz.....34
Drink Lots of Fluids.....35
Are You Dehydrated?.....35
What's Up with Vitamins and Supplements?.....37

Vitamins and Minerals: How You Get Them.....41
The Scoop on Supplements.....42

Section 4
Diets 43

The Protein Diet.....45
The Counting Calories Diet.....51
The Count Begins.....55
Setting Goals.....57
Being Aware of Calories.....58
A Low-Fat Approach.....59
Cholesterol in Foods.....62
Fat-Free Food Frenzy.....64
Pros to Low-Fat Eating.....65
Vegetarians.....66
The Pros and Cons of Being a Vegetarian.....69
Surviving as a Vegetarian.....72
Sugar Free.....74
The Plan.....75
Diet Fads.....77
What's Out There Today.....80
Words of Warning and Wisdom.....81
Avoiding the Weight Yo-Yo.....82
Our Own Approach.....83

Section 5
Fitness 89

Exercise.....91
Exercise + Dieting = Much Better Success.....95
What Is a Perfect Ten?.....95
Cardiovascular Fitness.....98
Cardiovascular a.k.a. Aerobic Exercises.....98

Strength Training.....106
Muscle Gain vs. Weight Loss.....112
Lifetime Fitness.....114
Perfect Exercises for Every Stage of Life.....117

Section 6
Cooking Healthy 119

Food Consciousness.....121
Ordering and Eating.....124
Eating at Home.....124
Healthy Recipes.....126

Section 7
Attitudes Toward Food 139

More Than a Swoosh.....141
Weighing Down with Weigh Down.....148
Eating Disorders.....150

Section 8
Reengineer Your Whole Life 157

Forming Habits That Help.....159
Dieting with Another Person.....166
The Parental Pass.....175
Life 101.....176

Introduction

So you're the chairman of the clean-plate club, but you'd rather not have so much to show for it. Living in an "I want it, and I want it yesterday" type of society sure doesn't make it easy on dieting folks. Dieting can be slow, frustrating, and downright confusing. Grab the bagel and hold the cream cheese or forsake all in the favor of a T-bone steak? Weight Watchers, Slim-Fast, Jenny Craig, or Richard Simmons?

Never fear, discerning digesters! This is the book for you. For within these pages waits all the information you'll ever need (at least for a while) to untangle the dieting dilemma. Simple explanations of the current diet trends and exercise options; health tips for the whole family; yummy and healthy (it can be done!) recipes are all included, as well as a big dose of encouragement.

We're not promising you instant six-pack abs, or that you'll fit into that little black dress by tomorrow, but we promise a book full of clues to the lifelong care and health of your incredible God-given body. Specifically, you'll find:

CATCH A CLUE

A Truckload of Clues. You'll learn tips from people who have lost weight and kept it off. You'll learn how they did it and why they've been so successful in the battle against the bulge.

WIDE ANGLE

Perspective. It's easy to get caught up in the daily trials of trying to lose weight. To be the most successful in the long run, though, we sometimes need help looking at the big picture. We'll help you take a step back.

WOW!

Humorous Stories. As worrisome as it can be, dieting does have its lighter side. We've collected a few choice stories for you.

DON'T FORGET

Important Reminders. Certain things are important to remember as you're dieting. We've highlighted those for you.

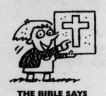

THE BOTTOM LINE

The Bottom Line. We'll help you get beyond confusion by letting you know the most important stuff to remember.

THE BIBLE SAYS

Help from Above. We've highlighted a few key Bible verses that will encourage you during your dieting woes.

Before you start yet another diet, you've got to do one thing: Read this book! It will save you a lot of frustration and confusion. Feel free to read it your way: from cover to cover or skipping around to the parts that interest you most. No matter how you read it, you'll find it's jammed with good advice, great ideas, and entertaining thoughts. So turn the page and start reading. . .you'll be glad you did!

Section 1
Warm Welcome to All Dieters

Cliff Divers Wanted

You're standing at the edge of a long, high cliff. All your friends are standing behind you, cheering you on.

"Jump, you wimp! Jump!"

You've only been cliff diving, for, well, you've never really been cliff diving. But you had a real good teacher. And, you've bought all the best equipment. Sweat beads form on your forehead. Your knees are getting weaker with each beat of your heart. The pinky on your right hand begins to twitch. The twitch quickly turns to a convulsive shake that takes over your whole body.

Then, you feel a hand on your back. Relief! Comfort! Security! You've felt this feeling before. You know exactly what to do. "Yes, God! Thank You for helping me in this moment of my need. Please protect me and deliver me from diving off this cliff." Feeling comforted, you relax and begin to turn around. You feel okay now. You don't have to jump.

But, it wasn't God's hand on your back. It was your friend. And she just pushed you off the cliff.

AAAAAAHHHHHHHHH!!!

Welcome to the wonderful world of dieting. Someone pushing you into the experience? Feeling pushed to lose some weight? Reshape your body? Get a little healthier? Whatever your reasoning, starting (or restarting) a diet can feel like jumping off a cliff. It's scary. It's difficult. But once you've accomplished your goal, you've conquered something unbelievable.

> **What's the Most Important Part of Dieting?**
>
> **THE BOTTOM LINE**
>
> It's starting. Starting your diet might feel almost impossible. And, the first few hours or days can be difficult. So, set a date and a time to start your diet, then commit to hold to it. Then, commit to not let go of it, to stay committed, and lose the weight you want.

HERE'S A HUG

We want this book to encourage you. Dieting shouldn't feel like a free fall off Mount Everest. You don't need to feel alone or desperate for advice. These pages contain a lot of information and, hopefully, a lot of encouragement. We've assembled all of this stuff because your diet is important. And, you need to succeed.

Welcome, Newbies!

Before you begin, we'd like you to try something.

First, go and get all of your recent junk mail and tear it up into small itty-bitty pieces. Next, tape-record yourself saying things like, "Congratulations! Way to go! Go get 'em! You'll come out a winner!" over and over. Finally, find three or four close friends (if you don't have friends, consider using good-looking strangers. If you aren't married, consider using *very* good-looking strangers!) who won't mind high-fiving you a few times. Got it? Great!

Now (timing is everything for this next step) play the tape you've created, toss the confetti you've made, and start high-fiving people.

There. Now you're ready to start your diet. Right?

Well, not really. If you've never dieted before, you're in for a treat. Let's just say, you're in for a treat—without treats, of course. Consider what's ahead of you.

GETTING HEALTHIER

Stop and think about what you're heading into here. Here are some possible synonyms for the phrase "getting healthier." Circle the one that best describes your intentions: cleaning house, getting organized, tuning up, looking better, just eating right.

Write a few of your own:

✓ into wt loss, ↓ cholesterol
try to get thyroid back in
control, ↓ glyco hemoglobin

However you phrase it, whatever you want to call what you're doing with your diet, you're getting healthier. And, getting healthier is a good thing. Why is getting healthier a good idea? Well, consider that your weight, or your diet, probably won't be an issue later in life if you begin to pay attention to it now. And, consider that you'll be able to do common tasks more easily if you're careful about what you eat.

So, first things first. You're getting healthier. And that's a good thing.

THE ALMIGHTY GOAL

Setting a goal, and then actually meeting it can make you feel like you've discovered some new bacteria and had it named after yourself. Accomplishing a goal can give you the feeling of fulfillment. But, setting a goal and not meeting it can make you feel rotten. There's nothing worse than setting out to accomplish something, then feeling like a failure when you miss the goal.

What you're learning in dieting can be much more than the right foods to eat or what exercise is best for you. You're learning about setting goals. You're learning about how to accomplish something that feels monumental.

Before you begin your diet, commit to yourself that you'll stick with this. On the lines below, write out your commitment. You may want to write out a sentence like, "I promise to keep this diet no matter what. And, if I am not able to fulfill this commitment to myself, I will seek out others who will be able to support me if I choose to try this again."

I need this diet so much! My weight is so out of weck!

Nothing in my life seems out of control esp: my dieting efforts.

A Rockin' Appearance

Let's not forget one of the reasons you might be dieting. It's no secret that many people diet so they'll look better in their favorite bathing suit, their wedding dress, or for a reunion. We want you to feel comfortable with desiring a better appearance. But, remember that you've got to love who you are before you diet, if you're going to love who you are after.

On the lines below, write out some words that describe your motivation for what you're about to attempt.

My weight, my lack of sustenance when it comes to dieting.

The result of all of this? You'll be looking better. You'll be feeling better. You'll be able to approach life with the satisfaction that you've set and met a goal.

WELCOME BACK!!

If you've tried dieting before, this time around might feel more like a trip to the dentist than an opportunity for growth, change, and a healthier lifestyle. Chances are, if you're trying this dieting thing again, it's because your previous diet halted abruptly. Maybe it stopped when you met your goal (yeah!), or when you couldn't resist that bag of popcorn at 1:00 A.M., or when you went on that three-week Coke and potato chip binge.

Whatever your reasoning, welcome back. Glad to have you. Before you launch your ship into the dieting waters, there's some advice we'd like to pass on to you.

YOU CAN DO IT!!

Say that title with us a few times. You CAN do it. It takes a lot to trim or change your eating and exercise habits.

Believe us when we tell you (like you need us to tell you this)—

others have been where you are. They've dieted, only to give in or give up. They've begun the fight, only to get knocked out in the first round. They've started their trek over the mountain, only to get driven back by a pack of wild dogs. They've—well. . .you get the point.

Just remember that others *have* had their diets interrupted by any number of factors, only to begin again, beat the odds, and hit their desired weight. Think through the things that might bring your diet to an abrupt halt. Write out some of them below so you'll remember to keep watch for them.

When my weight begins to go ↑ again, I feel defeated.

REFUSE THE FAKE OUT

If you're like many people, you began dieting with a bunch of false impressions. Maybe you've heard yourself saying things like:

- "I'm just a little overweight. I can conquer this weight thing in no time."
- "I can change my eating habits at the drop of a hat."
- "I'm not addicted to chocolate. Really!"
- "Breakfast is the most important meal of the day. That's why I eat three of them."

If you've said these things to yourself, watch out. Lying to yourself is the first sure sign of failing in your diet. So be honest.

Now is a good time to assess what you've done in the

THE BIBLE SAYS

In Control

The apostle Paul knew what it meant to be in control. He also knew what it was like to feel totally helpless. However you feel about your diet, let his words comfort you:

" 'My grace is sufficient for you, for my power is made perfect in weakness.' Therefore I will boast all the more gladly about my weaknesses, so that Christ's power may rest on me" (2 Corinthians 12:9).

past and why it didn't work. Take a moment and write down your previous dieting experiences.

Weight Watchers, First Place (a biblical one) + now ADA (1800 cal) diet

Now, look over your story. What tripped you up? Notice any previously unnoticed weak areas?

REMEMBER THIS!

We serve a God who gives us strength to make it, go for the goal, and complete every task we're called to. As you head into your diet, remember that God is with you. He made you. He knows you. He loves you just the way you are. And, He's helping you with what you're about to do! Cheers!

WOW!

Airplanes and Diets

Jean Kerr, author and playwright, says this about dieting:

"I feel about airplanes the way I feel about diets. It seems to me that they are wonderful things for other people to go on."

AMEN

What Do You Want?

EXAMINING YOUR MOTIVES

So why *do* you want to be on a diet?

OK, nobody *wants* to diet. Then why do you believe that you *need* to be dieting? What is it you want to accomplish? What is it you think you need to change? What is your motivation?

The way we feed ourselves is a pattern that intertwines with so many other parts of our lives. Losing weight is about our bodies, but it is also about our social customs and our patterns for nurturing ourselves and others. It's also about our need to please and our ability to wield power in a body-conscious society.

So why do *you* want to be on a diet? Finish this sentence. . .

"I need to diet because. . ."

_____

_____

If you have more than three reasons, don't list them all. Instead, prioritize the top three. Now answer this question using those three reasons:

"By dieting, I want to accomplish. . ."

_____

_____

_____

Dieting is not just food management. It is changing the way you live. That's hard to do. It's a lot of effort. It's hard to maintain at best, and particularly hard if you don't have a firm grasp on why you are making this change. Here are some of the most common reasons people go on diets:

• My doctor told me to.
• I want to look good for my reunion.
• My spouse wants me to.
• I want to feel better about myself.

- I want my husband to be proud of me.
- My joints are aching.
- I can't fit into any of my clothes, and I don't have the money to buy more.
- I feel ashamed.
- My mother-in-law suggested it.
- I want to wear a bathing suit this summer.
- I am a health risk to myself.
- I want firmer _____ (list body part).

Can you add a few more?

- _____

- _____

- _____

Our motivations for dieting are usually not much different from our motivations for anything else.

- ***We either do it for ourselves or we do it for others.***
  This is an important distinction. Whether we are trying to please a spouse, a parent, or a society, many of us diet for reasons that have nothing to do with our own selves; we are just trying to please. What we often don't realize is what that really means is that we are trying to change other people's attitudes by changing ourselves. We are try-ing to make them feel differently about us. Haven't we learned by now that, in the end, we can only change ourselves? It's OK to admit that you are losing weight for someone else, but take some time to find the advantages for yourself as well.

- ***We either do it out of guilt or out of inspiration.***
  There is such a shame in our culture about being overweight. We feel guilty. We feel substandard. We start a diet out of those feelings. That is reality. But it's often not the most effective way to lose weight. It's easier to lose weight when we are on our own side. That means we are cheering for ourselves and wishing ourselves the best rather than beating ourselves over our collective heads with a food plan.

- *We either do it for our physical health or we do it for our esteem.*
  There is no way that your esteem is not affected by losing weight or
  by gaining it. But at some point, you have to consider more than just
  the outer image. What is happening to your health as you carry this
  weight? More importantly, are you keeping in mind that losing weight
  is not just so your pants will fit better, but because your whole body
  will have a better chance of
  survival?

It's important for you to
know why you are dieting,
because that is the only
thing that will keep you on
your food plan when everything inside of you is beg-
ging you to stop this work
of changing your patterns
and give yourself a break. At
that point, if you don't know
why you are dieting, or if
you still don't believe in
your reasons, then you've
got a problem.

So why are you thinking
about starting a diet?

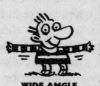

WIDE ANGLE

What Is Ten Pounds?

One dress size?
The mountain you
    can't get over?
The river you just
    can't cross?
A challenge? A race? A prize?
The weight of happiness?
The last step to perfection?
The closest you'll get to being happy
    with yourself?
The last thing you'll see before you
    celebrate?
What is ten pounds. . .to you. . .exactly?

Ranking Priorities

Just about everyone wants to look good. There's nothing wrong with wanting to look good. In fact, in our body-obsessed culture, it would be almost impossible not to be concerned with how your looks compare to the current ideal.

When you're considering the many reasons for dieting, though, looking good may not be the most important (or most effective) reason. Dieting is hard work. When you're in the midst of changing habits, saying no to yourself constantly, and altering life patterns, "looking good" is not a reason that will stick with you. And the real question is, what value is looking good if you don't take care of yourself and don't live a full life? Being healthy and living long are reasons for dieting that far outweigh the loss of inches and the new dress size.

That doesn't mean that you have to choose between reasons, but it means that you would do well to prioritize your reasons. When you hit the bumps in the road and want to quit, go down your list in the order of importance. Learn to care enough about yourself to take care of yourself, not just to impress other people. When you think about it, no matter how great you'll feel if you think you look good, that's still measuring yourself by other people's opinions. You know what? No matter how good you look, someone's still going to disapprove of something about you.

That's really the lie of the diet. We don't just think diets will change our weight; we think they'll change our lives. We think other people will treat us differently. We think a diet is the road to a new us, and often we are disappointed. Here's a secret about those beautiful people on the magazine covers...they are paid to smile and look good and look like their lives are all put together. It has nothing, neces- sarily, to do with reality.

WIDE ANGLE

Sweet Tooth or Salty Cravings?

Would you rather have a bag of salty popcorn or a candy bar?

Would you rather have a bowl of chicken and dumplings or blackberry cobbler with ice cream?

Would you rather have a turkey dinner with stuffing or pecan pie instead?

Would you rather have bread pudding or banana pudding?

You probably already know whether you crave sweet or salty things more. The real test is, what are you going to do about it?

Going on a diet may make your body smaller, or at least better shaped, but be careful what you wish for. If you are losing weight so other people will treat you differently or so your whole life will be better—here's a news flash—your body isn't where your well-being resides. You can make your life better by losing weight, but you won't fix your broken heart or your lost soul. Diets improve you, but they don't save you and they don't rescue you.

So while it will be great to look wonderful for the high school reunion or the new job, take some time to think about how you can take care of yourself by losing weight. What kind of investment do you want to make in your own life? Are you interested in giving yourself the longest life that is within your power to give? Do you want to be healthy and active for as long as you can? Do you want to enable yourself to have a positive outlook because you basically feel good? Losing weight can't guarantee you all these things. But you can surely have a better chance at them.

So take a look at your priorities in trying to "lose those unwanted pounds." A little thought now can help you last through this challenge because you know why you started and why you want to finish.

Recognizing Weaknesses

If losing weight was easy, everyone would be doing it. That's true for most of life, but especially for losing weight. Working off pounds is difficult in every way. It's difficult physically, because sooner or later it takes some exercise. It's difficult emotionally, because most of us have to find some new comfort besides the sweets and the starches. It's difficult mentally because you have to plan and prepare rather than just to the fast-food drive-thru when you feel like it. The list goes on and on. And no matter how many diet books tell you to concentrate on the "do's" and not the "don'ts," a diet with a purpose to shed pounds is a diet that has some "don'ts" in it. Every "don't" makes the whole plan that much more difficult.

One of the keys of successful dieting is recognizing your own "don'ts." It's knowing what your particular weaknesses and soft spots are, no matter which particular food plan you are sticking to. Does it seem impossible to go to bed without that evening snack? Does the sweet tooth overtake you every afternoon? Does it just feel too hard to do without that biscuit on the way to work? Is it the salty foods or the sweet ones? Is it a certain time of day? Is it boredom? Depression? Family holidays? All of the above?

Knowing where your weaknesses are can help you prepare for them. Not recognizing those soft spots leaves you vulnerable to the same mistakes over and over and over again.

Once you know your cravings, then, a real key to success is finding the least harmful way to give in to yourself a little. From finances to food, the experts will tell us that few of us find success if we deny ourselves everything we want. Usually we are just setting ourselves up for a fall. So how can you cater to yourself a bit without blowing it completely? Craving pizza? Many grocery store delis sell pizza by the slice now. You don't need to buy a whole pizza to have a taste. Want a burger and fries? Make a turkey burger and oven-bake some thinly-sliced potatoes. Get creative. Get crazy. Meet your cravings head-on and plan ahead to give in, but with control.

Setting Realistic Goals and Time Frames

We want it now. No, we want it yesterday. In our modern culture we can often get what we want quickly. But dieting just doesn't work that way. Our bodies will not be hassled or hustled by us without consequences. If we don't have a long-term plan to support the short-term effort, then we can become yet one more dieting casualty.

Who hasn't heard it? It took you a long time to put on the weight, and it will take you a long time to take it off. As true as this may be, it's almost always an unwanted comment.

Most weight loss experts agree that two pounds a week is a realistic maximum for regular, consistent weight loss. Most will also admit that to do that without a plateau here and there is almost impossible. You can do the math. That's about eight pounds a month on a good month. That means that when you spend seven long days fighting cravings and saying no to yourself and then you get on the scales and it's just two marks lower than last week—that's good news.

But that two pounds seems like a small payoff for the dailiness of it all, doesn't it? Settle it for yourself. That's what it takes.

If thirty pounds is what you want to lose, then give yourself at least four months to lose it. If you don't have four months before your deadline, change your goal. The only thing worse than not losing the weight is losing it and then gaining it right back. Then you really *have* wasted your time and your energy and your willpower.

Why do we set unrealistic goals? Sometimes it's because we want that end result, and we think we can make our lives be only about that. The truth is, though, that our lives are about more than our bodies and our weight. Stresses or tragedies come that sidetrack us. Vacations and people come into our lives and

What If. . .

If I woke up tomorrow and was my ideal weight, I'd call me up a feller and I'd ask him for a date.

WOW!

If I woke up tomorrow and I was nice and thin,
I'd dress me up real pretty and even show some skin.
If I woke up tomorrow to scales with real good news,
I'd take me out that evening to any place I choose.
But if I wake up tomorrow, same as I am today,
I'd just as well quit waiting and do it all anyway.

disrupt our exercise schedules. Illness or accidents step in unexpectedly. We have to remember that our "best" is the best we can do given our whole lives and our specific situations.

Unrealistic goals feel good when we set them. We can sometimes feel almost superhuman. But they don't work, and the other side of the coin is that we feel like a failure when we aren't. We feel like we've let someone down by not accomplishing the goal, when we really let ourselves down by setting the goal.

Be fair to yourself. Really count the cost and know what your goals will require of you. You are an intelligent person. Don't expect more than it's possible to give. That way you're giving yourself a chance.

Section 2
What to Expect

Overview of the Book

You've decided it's time to slim down and get into shape, but there is so much conflicting information on dieting and fitness out there that it's anyone's guess where to start. Well, you've come to the right place. Think of this book as a mini tour through the world of dieting and fitness, and we are your guides, helping you make wise, informed decisions. The first stop includes healthy eating followed by a look at different diets and ways to change your eating habits. At our second stop you'll learn how to get in shape and decide how to go about it. Our third stop helps you develop healthy attitudes toward food, while the final stop shows you how to pass healthy eating and exercise habits on to your family.

How This Book Is Organized

This book has eight major parts, and each part is divided into chapters. Although you could pick up the book and read a part or chapter, we recommend reading the whole book to get a well-rounded look at dieting and fitness. Typical chapters include:

• Setting goals for calorie consumption
• How much fat you need in your diet
• Vegetarian cooking
• The benefits of exercise
• Toning versus strength training
• Healthy recipes
• Biblical principles toward food
• Helping your kids develop good life habits

It's Hard Work—Not a Miracle

If losing weight and getting in shape were easy, you wouldn't need this book. You may feel like you need a miracle to get back to your ideal weight, but it will only happen with lifestyle changes and a lot of hard work on your part. But don't let that scare you. Instead of adopting the "poor me; I can't eat what I want" attitude, think about putting yourself first. "I like me, and I'm going to take good care of me" is the attitude to adopt. This means eating low-calorie foods that are rich in valuable nutrients. Learn what foods you like within this category and eat them often. Find some activities you like and do them as often as possible.

Adopting these attitudes and incorporating exercise may be a whole new world to you, but don't be shy. Take it slow, and you'll find you actually like how you feel!

REFOCUS

It is easy to let food dominate our thoughts, but the Bible is pretty clear on how God feels about gluttony.

"If you are a big eater, put a knife to your throat" Proverbs 23:2 (NLT).

Now the Bible isn't literally saying to go kill yourself if you overeat, but it is pointing out that overeating is a serious problem that needs attention. While the Bible condemns gluttony, God has also provided food for us to enjoy.

"Eat your food. . .with a happy heart, for God approves of this!" Ecclesiastes 9:7 (NLT).

Let's keep the right attitude toward food. It is for our nourishment and sustainment. It is a gift from God.

RECOMMENDATIONS AND DISCLAIMERS

Before getting started, we recommend you take a look at your eating habits and examine why you eat the way you do. Take a look at the following list and determine if you find yourself eating because of these reasons:

Ever Think About This?

THE BIBLE SAYS "Whatever you eat or drink or whatever you do, you must do all for the glory of God" (1 Corinthians 10:31 NLT).

- **Boredom.** Do you often find yourself with nothing better to do, so you make and eat a sandwich or scarf a bag of chips or see how many green M&Ms are in the bag? Eating to keep your mind preoccupied will load up calories and put on weight in no time.
- **Moods.** Does this sound like some of your self-talk? "I think a chocolate chip cookie will put me in a better mood." Or, "I'm having a bad day. I deserve an ice cream sundae." Or, "That police officer didn't

give me a ticket! I'll celebrate with a candy bar." Eating with your moods usually means you'll be eating all of the time.

- *Childhood Habits.* How you were raised plays a huge role in how you eat now. If you were allowed to eat lots of candy and junk food, it's a good bet you still do. Maybe your mom didn't cook much, so you ate a lot of prepared foods. If you were raised in the South, you probably got used to rich, high-fat foods that taste wonderful but aren't healthy. Examine your growing-up years and identify how and what you ate.

- *Emotional Reasons.* Many people eat in response to stress—stress in their marriage, job, or family. Are you eating to take your mind off a problem you're dealing with? Do you find comfort in food (which you're not getting elsewhere in your life)? Do you eat when you're upset or angry? Identifying your stressors and finding alternative ways to deal with them will give your body a chance to listen and respond appropriately to your internal cues of hunger.

Behavioral Change

In order to lose weight, we recommend that you make a behavioral change. Yeah, you might have to change the foods that you eat or the portion sizes, but if you want the weight to stay off forever, you have to change the behaviors that surround your eating.

1. *Control the stimulus that causes you to overeat.*
   a. Shop from a list.
   b. Don't shop when you're hungry.
   c. Keep healthy foods in the front of the refrigerator.
   d. Use smaller plates when eating.

2. *Alter your eating behavior.*
   a. Chew food slowly and thoroughly.
   b. Do nothing while eating, like reading or watching TV.
   c. Pause in the middle of the meal.
   d. Stop eating before you feel full. The feeling of fullness comes twenty minutes after you've finished eating.

3. *Reward yourself for good behavior.*
   a. Plan specific rewards for specific behaviors.
   b. Family and friends can provide praise and material awards.

4. *Monitor yourself.*
Keep a diary that includes:
a. Time and place of eating.
b. Type and amount of food.
c. How you feel.

DISCLAIMER

This book is no guarantee that you are going to lose weight and get in shape. It is *all* up to you. We have provided the information, but you have to put it into practice. Just remember when you're feeling unmotivated that eating healthy and staying in shape are two of the most important things you can do for yourself. They have a huge impact on your current and future health and can mean the difference between enjoying your old age or needing long-term care. For whatever reason, whether it's lack of time, energy, or discipline, don't neglect your responsibility to keep yourself healthy.

Section 3
Nutrition

The Classic Food Pyramid

REMEMBER THE FOOD PYRAMID?

Wipe away the cobwebs and think back to the good ol' days of elementary school. Remember learning about the food pyramid, the symbol of the ideal American diet? Well, it's still around, believe it or not. While fad diets will always come and go, the food pyramid will remain constant. Maybe it's because it's well-constructed like the Egyptian pyramids. From the bottom up, the food pyramid consists of four levels. The solid base level of breads and cereals supports the entire pyramid, followed by the vegetables, fruits level, upon which rests the protein level, including meats and dairy products. The top level, the very tip of the pyramid, includes fats, oils, and sweets. Is it starting to come back to you? Back in school this was probably just something you learned for a grade, but now it pays to remember how many servings from each group you need on a daily basis.

DON'T FORGET

TILT!

Some foods fall into more than one group. For example, doughnuts may be considered in the bread group, but they are so high in fat they can be considered in the miscellaneous group. Eat foods such as pretzels, sweet rolls, and cream cheese sparingly. They can cause your food pyramid to become top-heavy and tip right over.

For the adult, the recommended number of servings from the breads and cereals, vegetables, fruits, dairy products, and meat group is four, three, two, two, and two, respectively. No servings are given for the fat group as these foods are not recommended and usually find their way into one's diet anyway. If this information is still a bit fuzzy in your brain, read on.

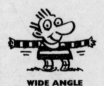

WIDE ANGLE

Pyramid

Breads and cereals: 4 servings

Vegetables: 3–5 servings

Fruits: 2–4 servings
Protein: 2 servings
Dairy products: 2–3 servings
Vegetables: 3–5 servings
Fats, oils, sweets: consume sparingly

Pyramid Contents

While it doesn't take a background in construction to build a healthy meal out of the pyramid materials, knowing which foods fit into what categories helps. Let's take a little tour of each food group.

Bread and Cereal Group: This food group includes bread and cereals (obviously), rice, pasta, grains, tortillas, pancakes, muffins, bagels, and cornbread.

Vegetable Group: Carrots, corn, peas, broccoli, spinach, sweet potatoes, Brussels sprouts, cabbage, cauliflower, squash, green beans, collard greens, lettuce, mushrooms, beets, and peppers. Be sure to eat some of each color.

Fruits: Everyone knows about apples, pears, plums, grapes, bananas, and peaches. But don't forget about grapefruit, nectarines, strawberries, blueberries, raspberries, apricots, prunes, dates, and the more exotic fruits such as kiwi, star fruit, ugli fruit, papaya, and mango.

Meat and Meat Alternatives: Poultry, beef, fish, pork, lamb, beans, eggs, peanut butter, dried peas and tofu, nuts, and seeds.

Dairy Products: Milk, soy milk, dry milk, cheese, cottage cheese, buttermilk, yogurt, custard, and ice cream.

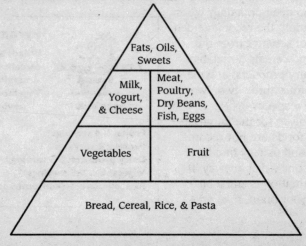

BALANCE CHECK

If you were to build a food pyramid out of the foods you ate yesterday, would it be so out of balance that it wouldn't even stand? Some people find that they are eating way too much from one food group and not enough of another group. If you're typical, you like to eat fast food. Unfortunately, a hamburger, fries, and milk shake, while it seems to be a good mix from the bread, meat, and dairy groups, contains so much fat that your pyramid will be too heavy and topple right over. Or maybe you like to eat a fifteen-ounce steak which weighs in at five times the amount of protein you should eat for the entire day! Is the only dairy you consume an ice-cream sundae before going to bed? Does the thought of eating veggies bring back bad memories of your parents making you sit at the table until you finished them, so now you refuse? All of these scenarios are examples of imbalanced eating which can result in obesity and a lack of essential nutrients. So do a balance check on your eating habits and make adjustments where necessary.

On My Own. . .

CATCH A CLUE

"When I moved into my own apartment, I never cooked vegetables and rarely ate any fruit. After several months I started to feel sluggish and gained quite a bit of weight. It wasn't until a friend at work pointed out that it might be because my diet was so imbalanced that I did something about it. Now that I eat some fruit and veggies every day, I feel so much better and have actually started to lose a few of those pounds."

—Carolyn, Hanover, Indiana

Count Your Servings

Take a look at the following serving sizes. You might be surprised to find how much you're really eating.

Breads and Cereals:
You should be eating four servings a day.
1 Serving = 1 slice of bread, 1/2 to 3/4 cup cooked cereal, rice, or pasta, 3/4 cup ready-to-eat cereal, 1 small potato, 1 large tortilla, 1/2 bagel

Meats:
You should be eating two servings a day.
1 Serving = 1 egg, 1/2 cup beans, 2 tablespoons of peanut butter, 1/4 cup nuts or seeds, or 2–3 ounces cooked chicken, poultry, meat, or fish Three ounces of meat is about the size of a deck of cards.

Vegetables:
You should be eating three to five servings a day.
1 Serving = 1 wedge lettuce, 1/2 cup carrots, 1/2 cup greens, 1/2 cup beets

Fruits:
You should be eating two to four servings a day.
1 Serving = 1/2 cup applesauce or 1 apple, 1/2 grapefruit, 1/2 banana, 1/2 cup orange juice

Dairy Products:
You should be eating two to three servings a day.
1 Serving = 1 cup milk or yogurt, 1/4 cup Parmesan cheese, 2 cups cottage cheese, 1 1/2 cups ice milk, 1 1/2 ounces cheese

Fats, Oils, Sweets:
No serving sizes are provided, as these find their way into the diet as ingredients in prepared foods.

So how does your daily diet weigh in? Are you eating a variety of foods and sticking to the serving sizes the food pyramid calls for? If not, now is the time to get in gear.

Don't Forget Your Fruits and Veggies!

"I'M POPEYE THE SAILOR MAN! I EAT LOTS OF SPINACH!"

He made spinach look like it tasted great! And what kid didn't want to be big and strong like Popeye? I remember thinking if eating spinach could do that for him, maybe it would make me a faster swimmer. So I asked my mom if she'd make some. Pleased as punch, she cooked up a batch,

WOW!

Top Five Most Hated Veggies of All Time

5. Asparagus
4. Beets
3. Sweet potatoes
2. Spinach
1. Brussels sprouts

but despite my high hopes, it was pretty hard to choke down. I decided being a fast swimmer wasn't worth that much. And so it goes with most kids. Veggies just don't taste good, and sometimes as adults our taste buds never turn around. Fruits don't get such a bad rap because they're a little sweeter, but most people still are not eating enough fruit a day to get their recommended daily allowance of vitamin C.

Eat Your Veggies!

Stuck in a rut and need some creative ways to incorporate more vegetables into your diet? The following ideas just might turn your whole world of vegetables around.

1. Eat raw, cut vegetables with your lunch. Dip them in some low-fat dip, and you have a healthy replacement for chips. In a rush? Buy the precut veggies at the grocery store, or cut a batch ahead of time and keep in baggies in the refrigerator. Carrots, broccoli, cauliflower, and peppers work best.

2. Have a salad. Add a variety of cut vegetables to dark green lettuces and spinach and voila! You have a healthy side to any meal. Be sure to use a low-fat dressing. In a rush? Buy the bagged salads. They tend to be skimpy on added vegetables, so add some precut veggies.

3. Serve mixed vegetables. Almost as healthy as fresh, frozen veggies are the next best thing. Often picked and immediately frozen, they retain many of their nutrients. So try heating a medley of veggies for some variety. Canned veggies are better than no veggies, but they tend to be high in salt. Buy the no- or low-salt versions and mix different ones together for some diversity.

4. Grill your vegetables. Skewering them works great and keeps them from falling in between the bars of the grill. Brush with a vinaigrette of olive oil and Worcestershire sauce and throw them on the grill. In a rush? You can buy pre-skewered veggies at most grocery stores.

5. Add cut vegetables to casseroles and spaghetti sauce.

6. Ask people for their favorite vegetable recipes. Sometimes you just need to get some new ideas from those you know and trust.

Feeling Fruity?

You've heard it a million times, "An apple a day keeps the doctor away." But believe it or not, one apple is not enough! The food pyramid calls for at least two servings of fruit a day. So somehow you're going to have to finagle another fruit into your diet. Read on for ideas.

Fit for Dogs

WOW!

"I remember my mom frequently making me sit at the dinner table until I finished my vegetables. One evening I couldn't go out to play until I had eaten the fifteen peas (over and over I counted them) on my plate. But much to my advantage that night, our dog was under the table and she got her serving of vegetables for the day!"
—**Stephen, Tofte, Minnesota**

1. Start with breakfast. Add some banana to your cereal. Sprinkle some berries on your granola. Have half of a grapefruit. Try some applesauce with your pancakes. And no, fruit jelly on your toast doesn't count.

2. Snack on fruit. Have a handful of grapes or dried fruit when those hunger pangs hit in between meals. And if you're tired of that apple, try some strawberries or mango instead.

3. Sneak some fruit into your dessert. Try some strawberries on your ice cream. Make strawberry shortcake or baked apples. Even a fruit salad with a cookie is a nice light treat.

VARIETY SHOW

Just as man can't live on bread alone, nor can he live on celery and rice cakes alone. At some point, your mouth and body will rebel. Not only will your taste buds get bored, you will actually get hungry sooner than if you had

THE BOTTOM LINE

Vitamin Supplements

Vitamin supplements are no match for the real foods they replace and should not be used in place of eating healthy meals that include fruits and vegetables. Don't choose a pill over real food.

eaten a regular meal. And what's the normal response to hunger between meals? Snacking. And because your taste buds are dying for something tasty, you end up snacking on high-fat/low-nutrient foods. Watch out for those vending machines!

Health Issues

If this sounds like you, don't be fooled into thinking that it's OK to snack on candy bars and chips because you're eating celery and rice cakes during the rest of the day. It only takes six to eight weeks to develop deficiencies in the B vitamins, thiamin, and riboflavin! If you're not eating a variety of foods, you won't get the nutrients you need, and your health will suffer. Energy levels will dwindle, mental alertness will dull, and all you will be able to focus on will be what you're going to eat next.

THE BOTTOM LINE

Health Risks

Not eating a variety of food poses real and life-threatening problems that are no laughing matter. Here is a list, to name a few:
Osteoporosis
Cancer
Heart disease
Hypertension
Diabetes
Infertility

Different Choices

Stuck in the rut of eating the same meals every night of the week? Take a few pointers from our test kitchen and add a little spice to your dinner fare.

- Alternate meatless meals with ones that contain meat.
- Learn to cook meats in a variety of ways: grilling, baking, broiling, stir-frying, etc.
- Experiment with fresh, frozen, and cut vegetables. Steaming veggies is a quick and nutritious way to cook them.
- Try some fruit-based desserts—apple crisp and berries on ice cream, for instance.

MENU IDEAS

Here's a skeleton list of dinners for five nights that you can detail to your own taste buds. But it will give you an idea of some healthy choices with a variety of tastes.

Day #1:
Fish—grilled or baked
Baked potato
Steamed vegetables topped with
    cheese

Day #2:
Pasta with sauce and added
    vegetables
Garlic bread
Fruit slices or salad

Day #3:
Chicken with rice casserole
Salad
Fresh bread

WIDE ANGLE

Caught Ya!

"Once a coworker of mine was on a diet and only ate grapefruit for breakfast; dry cereal, dried fruit, and a Diet Coke for lunch; and things like dry pasta, rice, and small amounts of chicken for dinner. But she never lost weight because she was always raiding the vending machines between meals for candy bars and chips!"
—Jana, Miami, Florida

Day #4:
Soup—there are several dry soups on the market that you add veggies
    and water to.
Crackers
Fruit slices

Day #5:
Mexican burrito with beans and rice
Raw, cut vegetables

Diet Quiz

Take this quiz to find out how varied your diet is.

1. How many times a day do you eat fruit?
    a. three
    b. two
    c. one
    d. none

2. How often do you eat veggies?
    a. five to seven days a week
    b. two to three days a week
    c. one day a week
    d. rarely

3. How often do you eat beef?
    a. once a week
    b. twice a week
    c. three to four times a week
    d. five or more times a week

4. How often do you eat fast food?
    a. rarely
    b. once a week
    c. two to three times a week
    d. four or more times a week

5. How many dairy products do you consume in a day?
    a. three
    b. two
    c. one
    d. none

KEY: A = 1 point. B = 2 points. C = 3 points. D = 4 points.
Add up your answers and see how your diet fares.
5–8 Keep up the good work.
9–12 Not bad.
13–16 You need some help.
17–20 It wouldn't kill you to eat an apple now and then!

Drink Lots of Fluids

Believe it or not, fifty-five to sixty percent of a person's body weight is water. It's so vital to our existence that even though one could go lengthy periods without food, he will survive only a few days without drinking water or fluids. In our body, fluids:

- Carry nutrients and waste products throughout the body.
- Fill the cells and the spaces between them.
- Serve as solvents for minerals, vitamins, and a multitude of other small molecules.
- Act as lubricants for joints.
- Serve as shock absorbers inside the eyes, spinal cord, and amniotic sac in pregnancy.
- Aid in body temperature regulation.

Fortunately the amount of fluid in our body is regulated to remain constant, but our systems are not perfect, and imbalances, such as dehydration, do occur.

Are You Dehydrated?

The average person loses two quarts of water a day just through daily living activities, while active people lose even more. Wondering how in the world you could be losing that much water every day? Well, in addition to the water excreted from your kidneys, you lose water through your lungs as vapor, through your feces and skin, and during the metabolism of the food you eat. So you need to be replacing that water daily. Unfortunately, many do not replace that water and are chronically dehydrated. While one usually thinks about dehydration as something that only people who exercise in the heat have to worry about, as you read this, you too are probably dehydrated to some extent. Dehydration is cumulative and will take its toll on those who fail to drink enough fluids on a regular basis. If you're waiting until you feel thirsty to drink, some dehydration has already started to occur. Thirst lags behind water lack, so when the mouth gets pasty and dry, promptly find the aqua. Serious dehydration can happen, especially in hot weather, for the gardener, the sunbather, and the exerciser.

DRINK HOW MUCH WATER?!

Yes, it's true. Since your body is losing two quarts of water a day, that means you have to drink two quarts of water a day to make up for it. And even more if you exercise! Don't worry, you won't be spending the entire day in the bathroom, but you should be making a few more pit stops. We know, you're wondering how in the world you're going to get that much water down, but never fear, we have a few pointers.

1. Break it down.

Two quarts equals sixty-four ounces. That breaks down to eight, eight-ounce glasses of water a day. Whew!! But drinking that much is definitely doable. If you like to be scheduled, try this pattern:

CATCH A CLUE

Dehydration Warning Signs:

- urinating small amounts of dark, yellow urine
- fatigue
- loss of appetite
- flushed skin
- light-headedness
- heat intolerance

- 8:00 A.M. or starting when you get up, drink eight ounces.
- 10:00 A.M., drink eight more ounces.
- 12:00 noon, drink another glass with lunch.
- 2:00 P.M., try eight ounces.
- 4:00 P.M., drink eight ounces with a snack.
- 6:00 P.M., drink eight ounces with dinner.
- 8:00 P.M., guzzle another eight ounces.
- 10:00 P.M. or before bed, drink a final eight ounces.

But I'll be getting up in the middle of the night to go to the bathroom! Then try drinking sixteen ounces with a lunch or dinner and skip the 10:00 glass.

2. What if. . .

If you're not that scheduled, try filling a two-quart container with water in the morning and then plan to have drunk the whole thing by the end of the day.

3. One final pointer

Jazz up your water with slices of lemon or lime. It seems to make the water a little more palatable. You can even put some in your two-quart container, and you're set for the day.

A WORD ABOUT JUICE

Juice is one way to consume some of the sixty-four ounces of daily needed water, but be careful in your juice choices. As you stroll down the drink aisle at the grocery store, bright colors and flavors catch your attention, but remember not all juice drinks are created equal. Many are called "fruit drinks" and contain very little juice but are filled with sugar. Some actually contain less than ten percent juice! Others, such as cranberry juice, are very high in calories. So be sure to read the label and limit your consumption. Water is always the best choice.

What's Up with Vitamins and Supplements?

VITAMINS AND MINERALS: WHAT THEY ARE AND WHY YOU NEED THEM

Our bodies (no matter what size they are) are pretty amazing. Everything works together: muscles, nerves, organs, cells, etc., etc., etc. We're usually aware of the obvious things that our bodies do to keep us alive, like our lungs breathing and our wounds healing. But there is so much that goes on at a level that we can't see. Our bodies are working all the time to keep us healthy.

One of the lesser known, but busier, elements of our bodies are our enzymes. Enzymes are catalysts in the constant chemical reactions that make up every breath we take, every meal we digest, and every voluntary and involuntary thing we do. The enzyme level is where vitamins and minerals first come into play.

Vitamins work with the enzymes in our body to help them do their jobs. Sometimes vitamins and minerals are even categorized as coenzymes because they work closely with and even (in some cases) activate enzymes. When we don't have enough vitamins and minerals in our bodies, we might have the enzymes we need, but they don't do the job we need them to do. We are then in a world of hurt.

Minerals also function as coenzymes, but they also become a part of our bodies (such as our bones and fluids) to keep us the right density (or texture) so that our blood will flow well and our bones will hold us up.

Besides helping our enzymes function and our bodies to maintain their consistency, vitamins and minerals help us in a lot of other ways. They keep the oxygen in our bodies clean and useful (antioxidants). In some cases they even affect our hormones or function as hormones themselves.

As you read about and look at vitamins and minerals, you'll hear the words "fat soluble" and "water soluble." Vitamins B and C are water-soluble vitamins. That means that they begin to be used by the body as soon as they are digested and they are flushed out of the body quickly. The other vitamins are "fat soluble." That means they become part of our bodies. They are absorbed into us. They leave at different rates, but much more slowly than vitamins B and C. With these kinds of vitamins, there can actually be a danger of overloading. Too much of one of them can function like a toxin in your body.

DON'T FORGET

Vitamin and Mineral Roll Call

Here's the skinny on some vitamins and minerals that you hear a lot about these days.

Vitamin/Mineral	Food Source	Benefits
Vitamin A and Beta Carotene	Green and yellow fruits and veggies, animal livers	Good for your eyes and skin, your immunity, and tissue maintenance
B Vitamins	Green leafy veggies, whole grains, proteins such as fish, chicken, turkey, eggs, beans	Good for your nervous system, stress relief, skin, and hair
Vitamin C	Green veggies, citrus fruit, berries	Good for immunity, growth and repair of your tissues, and even cancer prevention
Vitamin D	Saltwater fish, dairy products fortified with Vitamin D	Good for helping the body use calcium, immunity, and the treatment/prevention of osteoporosis.
Vitamin E	Dark green leafy veggies, nuts, beans, whole grains	Good for cardiovascular disease, circulation, PMS
Vitamin K	Green leafy veggies	Good for blood and bone formation
Folic Acid	Red meat, poultry livers, pork, green leafy veggies, whole wheat, yeast	Good for cells, relieving stress, helps metabolism

Calcium	Dairy foods, salmon, seafood, green leafy veggies	Good for bones, teeth, nervous system, and muscle function
Chromium	Meat, cheese, whole grains, brewer's yeast	Good for metabolizing glucose, diabetes, reducing cholesterol
Magnesium	Distributed in foods, particularly dairy, meat, and fish	Good for bones, nerves, muscles, energy, blood
Potassium	Dairy, poultry, fish, beans, whole grains	Good for blood pressure, energy, and hormones
Iron	Meat, fish, liver, eggs, green leafy veggies, whole-grain breads, cereals	Good for blood, energy, and immunity
Zinc	Seafood, especially oysters, whole grains, beans	Good for healing, taste, smell, immunity

Vitamins and Minerals: How You Get Them

You're *supposed* to get your vitamins and minerals from the food you take into your body. You can drink orange juice and get vitamin C. You can eat green leafy vegetables and get vitamins E and K. You can eat chicken livers and get vitamin A. You can eat sardines and get calcium or you can drink milk which will give you magnesium too. You can eat a banana (as a current TV commercial makes clear) and there's your potassium. The ideal plan is that through the meals you eat, your body receives the necessary vitamins and minerals.

The ideal plan worked better when our culture was more agrarian and slower paced. Nutrients weren't cooked out of foods and then replaced artificially. There weren't as many kinds of convenient, nutrition-deprived snacks.

CATCH A CLUE

What Is an Antioxidant?

If you read about vitamins for more than fifteen minutes, you're going to read about antioxidants.

If your body were a sci-fi movie, the bad guys would be the free radicals (dressed in black, of course). The good guys would be the antioxidants (in white, horses and all).

At the cellular level, oxygen molecules travel in pairs. When something stresses them, they split like a bad marriage. Each half of the oxygen team looks for something else to pair up with. That "other molecule" is a free radical. That pairing damages the integrity of your tissues, whether that means cataracts, wrinkles, diseases, arthritis, etc.

Antioxidants neutralize free radicals. Antioxidants set their phasers on kill and go about cleaning up the place. Without antioxidants, your free radicals would take over the planet that is called "Your Body." Many vitamins and minerals provide you with antioxidants. Read labels.

Unfortunately in our current cultural climate, foods are not as nutritious. More chemicals are used in their growth and preparation. Less foods are eaten whole. Instead they are processed (which basically means they have the nutrients beaten out of them). Because of this, we often supplement our diets with vitamin and mineral pills or with liquid nutrients like diet shakes.

The Scoop on Supplements

You might have heard. . .some people think you shouldn't take supplements. They say that you should get your vitamins and minerals the organic way: through the foods you eat. You might have also heard. . .some people think you should definitely take supplements. You might have also heard. . .some people who say you shouldn't take supplements do take supplements.

The reality is that we often don't eat what we should, even when it's available to us. And even when we give it a good effort, the foods that we eat don't always live up to their full potential. So we often supplement the nutrition we receive.

Nutrition supplements come in many forms.

- **Pills or tablets.** Vitamins and minerals come in the form of a pill that you take with water. Many herbals, such as Saint John's wort or garlic, come in that form as well. In this day and age you have a broad array of pill supplements in all combinations. Evaluate your needs and supplement away.

- **Liquid supplements.** Many liquid supplements are described with the term "shakes." To use the word "shakes" is a loose interpretation of these supplements. They are really canned milk-like drinks (or powder that you add to water or milk). You do shake them to make sure the nutrients in them (necessary for the chalky taste in some) are well-distributed, but to compare them to a milk shake is a big leap.

  Some shakes are particularly geared toward dieters and function as meal replacers (Slimfast, Success). Others are geared toward nutrition, particularly targeting seniors in their marketing (Assure). Yet another kind of liquid supplement is the fiber supplement that you mix with water (Metamucil, Citrucel).

- **Fruit bars**. In some cases, and particularly certain food plans, you can eat fruit-flavored bars to supplement your intake of vitamins and minerals in ways that don't require food. This helps the dieter to eat nutritiously while cutting calories.

Section 4
Diets

The Protein Diet

A MISNOMER? A DISCLAIMER?

There is a whole category of diets that is called high-protein diets. That's the way the bookstores categorize them on the shelves. That's the way the hip-hop diet gurus talk about them. For the most part, though, these diets are not so much high protein as they are low carbohydrate. When you read the best-sellers these diets are based on, you find as much written about starch and sugar as you do about protein.

So call them protein diets if you want, but keep in mind that what you do without is as significant as what you include on these food plans.

A LOOK AT THE CRAZE DR. ATKINS STARTED

Dr. Atkins was one of the first, if not *the* first, to stand up and say, *"It's not the fat that's making us fat! It's the sugar!"* Furthermore, he told us that it isn't just the white sugar on the table that is making us fat. It is the sugar that is made in our bodies when we eat starchy foods or carbohydrates, particularly refined flour.

In the seventies when Dr. Atkins's book, *Diet Revolution* was published, the trend toward low-fat foods had already begun. There were low-fat options on the horizon everywhere. Total fat intake was down throughout the country. Yet obesity was on the rise and diseases like heart disease and breast cancer were running rampant. These observations coupled with research convinced Dr. Atkins that fat was not the real culprit. As manufacturers had lowered the fat content in foods, they had raised the carbohydrate content, in particular simple carbohydrates:

THE BOTTOM LINE

How Many Carbs Is Too Many?

For most people, carbs should make up about forty percent of their diet. More than fifty percent could be a problem. That really sounds like a lot, doesn't it? But think of a plate with four ounces of meat, corn on the cob, mashed potatoes, and a roll. That's about seventy-five percent carbs. How about spaghetti noodles with sauce and a salad and rolls? That's more than fifty percent. Add in a sweet dessert, and you're well on your way to way too many carbs.

sugars. The more of these carbohydrates we ate the less likely we were to lose weight. Here is some of the research that supports Dr. Atkins's conclusions (from http://www.atkinscenter.com):

"If, as we had been told, heart disease results from the consumption of saturated fats, one would expect to find a corresponding increase in animal fat in the American diet. Actually the reverse is true. During the sixty-year period from 1910 to 1970, the proportion of traditional animal fat in the American diet plummeted from eighty-three percent to sixty-two percent, the proportion of butter consumption from eighteen pounds per person per year to four. During the past eighty years, dietary vegetable fat in the form of margarine, shortening, and refined oils increased about four hundred percent and the consumption of sugar and processed foods increased about sixty percent."
—Sally Fallon, *Nourishing Traditions*, 1995 Promotion Publishing

Dr. Atkins became the voice that asked us to get rid of sugars and to lower carbs and become healthier. Now if you get rid of sugars and lower your carbs, you're left with mostly protein and fiber, so Dr. Atkins's diet became known as the protein diet.

Even though Dr. Atkins spoke out against carbohydrates, he also outlined what some today suppose to be late-breaking news. He outlined the danger of the high insulin levels that are induced in our bodies by a high-carb food plan. There have been more and more doctors, researchers, and nutritionists since Dr. Atkins to echo his battle cry, but he was the first of note.

A Word from the Good Doctor Himself

Dr. Atkins says (http://www.atkinscenter.com) that there are three "wonderful" results from his food plan.

1. You'll start to burn fat for energy rather than the food you eat.
2. You won't feel hungry in between meals.
3. Your overall health will improve, and you'll feel better.

Much of the benefits of Dr. Atkins's food plan is based on his research on the villain, sugar. Dr. Atkins calls sugar an antinutrient since it causes your body to work without giving anything back. He states that the average person now consumes over 150 pounds of sugar a year, up from less then ten pounds in the nineteenth century. Check out this quote from a Johns Hopkins news release that Dr. Atkins includes with his web page:

"Johns Hopkins researchers have found evidence that some cancer cells are such incredible sugar junkies that they'll self-destruct when deprived of glucose, their biological sweet of choice. . . Scientists have long supected. . .the cancer cell's heavy reliance on glucose. . ."

Do you get the feeling that Dr. Atkins has done some homework and that maybe we should ask to cheat off of it?

Dr. Atkins calls white flour sugar's second cousin since it turns immediately to sugar in the body. This is why he rants and raves (on the written page) about the dangers of so many of our processed foods being made almost entirely out of refined white flour. The double danger is that we simply don't realize how much sugar we are eating because it's in the form of something unsweet, at least until it digests.

Success Stories

WOW!

For all its critics, the low-carb diet has plenty of success stories. You don't have to look farther than http:www.atkinscenter.com:

Christopher dropped 152 pounds and can wear his wedding ring again.

Tricia, in less than a year, went from a size 22 to a size 5.

Kathi claims Dr. Atkins's diet gave her her life back. She went from a size 18 to a size 6 in just six months.

Maura feels her success is almost too good to be true. Her husband lost eighty-five pounds (size 42 waist to a 30 waist), and she lost seventy-five pounds (size 18 to a size 4). People don't even recognize them.

Margaret says she's wearing her "skinny" clothes every day now!

Kathy calls this diet a beautiful gift and the easiest, most delicious way of eating that "makes me feel so good." She's lost forty-seven pounds.

Gail lost ninety-eight pounds. With Dr. Atkins's diet, her sugar, blood pressure, and cholesterol levels are normal. She loves this diet. She now has six coworkers following her example.

Despite all the criticism aimed at Dr. Atkins and his food plan (many of which are aimed at misunderstandings or characterizations)—it's hard to fight with success.

WHY NOT EAT CARBOHYDRATES?

Basically, carbohydrates (known by their friends as "carbs") are the quick-energy food. They are what the body uses first for energy. They are also what needs to be renewed most often. This is why (if you have any marathoners in your family, you probably know this) athletes often eat high-carb meals the night before a big event. They are loading up on the substances that will be most readily available to their body for energy the next day.

No matter what carbohydrate you eat, whether it's a candy bar or a potato, the first thing your body does is break it down into sugar. Sugar is the simplest form of carbohydrate. So whether it's cake or rolls or biscuits or Lifesavers, the first thing those foods do in your body is break down into sugar.

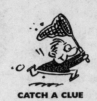

CATCH A CLUE

Hair Loss?
Your hair is made of protein. Did you realize that? The bad news is that low-protein diets are often the cause of hair loss in men and women. The good news is that this kind of hair loss is easily reversible by adding enough protein back into the diet.

Now apply that information to a dieter. The purpose of dieting is to take in less calories than your body needs so that it breaks into its fat storage for some of its energy. As it does that you lose weight. But if you are constantly filling your body with the first thing it'll reach for to get energy, when does it have the opportunity to start using up those fat storages? *It doesn't!* In fact, it probably stores more fat. That's why people can eat low-fat things and not lose weight—but instead even gain weight.

When you think about it, it's so simple you have to wonder why we don't realize what we are doing. We keep hearing people say, "Just because it's fat free doesn't mean you can eat as much as you want." Nevertheless we eat more of something when we know it's fat free because we feel like we're doing something good for ourselves.

WHY EAT PROTEIN?

Protein's primary function is to maintain and repair body tissue. When you don't have enough protein in your diet and thus in your body, cuts don't heal as quickly and injuries occur more often. That's because your bones and cartilage and basic tissue don't have enough of what makes them up (protein) to renew themselves.

When you are dieting, at least when you are dieting the low-carb way, your body goes looking for energy to maintain and repair itself. It first uses up the carbohydrates or sugars that are hanging around. If it doesn't find enough of those, it starts working on the proteins. If there aren't enough proteins from your food then your body will use whatever proteins it finds—like its own muscles and tissues. This is what we *don't* want to have happen. When you are using your own protein for living energy, you are not becoming more healthy; you are become mal-nourished. What we want the body to do is go for the fat storage. So (according to the low-carb people):

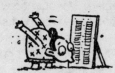

Protein Facts

THE BOTTOM LINE

- **Protein's role is to maintain and repair our tissues.**
- **It composes muscles, tendons, and ligaments.**
- **Protein is four calories per gram.**
- **It is used for energy in the absence of carbs.**

1. We rob our bodies of carbs so our bodies keep searching,
2. We give them enough protein so that they function without emaciating us, and
3. We exercise to put the extra *oomph* in there to chase our bodies to our fat cells to find energy.

Then we lose weight the right way. Our bodies are using up the extra that we've packed in instead of the nutrients we need to keep running.

Protein helps our bodies run efficiently in another way. There are minerals in our body that can be toxic or helpful (such as iron or copper). What makes the difference is whether they have enough protein to bond to. When these minerals (and others) bond to protein, the protein acts as a chaperone, carrying the minerals around our bodies to the places they are needed. When there is not enough protein in our bodies for this escort service to function, those same substances become free agents that can do damage at will.

Is It for You?

Of course you know that only you can answer that, with your physician's help, but there are a few things to consider. . .

Do you eat a lot of simple carbohydrates made of

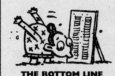

Quiz Time

THE BOTTOM LINE

What are the only foods that contain practically no protein?

Fruits, sugar, vegetable oils

sugar or refined white flour? What happens to you if you quit those foods for a few days? Can't make it without them for a few days?

How about a few meals? It would be worth your efforts to see.

There aren't a lot of negative risks on a low-carb (often called a high-protein) food plan. Just make sure, whether it is Atkins or Sugar Busters or whatever, that you aren't cutting out carbohydrates completely. Instead you should simply be substituting the most healthy, fiber-filled carbs for the sweets and refined white flour carbs.

Also, if you have a lot of fluctuations in your energy level, you might want to ask your doctor to check out your blood sugar levels and talk to you a bit about your carbohydrate intake. Often people who begin a low-carb plan uncover health problems that already existed but were masked by their high-carb intake. Better to know now than to blame a diet later for damage that has already been done.

The Counting Calories Diet

WHY COUNT CALORIES?

"I want to lose weight, but counting calories seems so time consuming," you say. It does take time, but it is well worth the effort to find out if you're eating more calories than you are expending each day—the main reason people gain weight.

Ever wondered why five years ago you weighed less than you do now, but nothing in your life has changed? It's because on a daily basis you've eaten a few more calories than you are burning, and over time these calories add up to be extra pounds. If the number of calories you eat is even with the number of calories you burn, you have an energy balance and will maintain your current weight. If your energy (calorie) intake is greater than your energy expenditure, then you will gain weight. The upside of counting calories is that it doesn't take long to learn how many calories are in different foods. So pretty soon you'll just be able to look at your meal and know approximately how many calories it contains.

How Much Protein Do You Need?

CATCH A CLUE

For most people who weigh about 150 pounds, two four-ounce servings per day are sufficient. Think of a four-ounce serving as the size of a deck of cards. You will get more from the protein you eat if you spread it across as many meals as possible instead of one huge steak at dinner.

COMMON CALORIE MISCONCEPTIONS

1. If I break the cookie into small pieces, it won't have as many calories.
2. I'll burn more calories if I chew fast.
3. A Diet Coke and French fries equal zero calories. They cancel each other out.
4. Cooking food helps reduce its calories.
5. If a food or drink is clear, it doesn't have any calories.

CALORIE QUIZ

Answer the following questions to find out how much you know about calories in common foods.

1. Which has more calories?
   A. an ounce of jelly beans
   B. an ounce of chocolate
2. Which has more calories?
   A. a slice of pound cake
   B. a slice of cheesecake
3. Which has fewer calories?
   A. a pound of peanuts
   B. a pound of M&Ms candy
4. Which has fewer calories?
   A. 1 cup of Parmesan cheese
   B. 1 cup of sour cream
5. Which has more calories?
   A. a Taco Bell Burrito Supreme
   B. a McDonald's hamburger

Key:
1. B; A = 104, B = 150
2. B; A = 110, B = 278
3. B; A = 2576, B = 2469
4. A; A = 455, B = 479
5. B; A = 257, B = 413

WIDE ANGLE

Where Does Protein Come From?

The following foods are good sources of protein:

Eggs	Fish
Milk	Nuts
Cheese	Beans
Meat	Whole-grain cereals
Poultry	Rice

CALORIES IN COMMON FOODS

It's always a little scary to find out the number of calories in your favorite foods. Sometimes we think what we don't know won't hurt us. Calories? What calories? Well, you know that handful of M&Ms candy you just ate? The calories didn't just melt in your mouth! To find the number of calories in foods you buy and prepare, read the labels. Bad eyesight? Get glasses. (There really are no excuses.) For other foods, check out a nutrition book from your library, or browse a local bookstore. Fast-food restaurants publish the calorie contents of their food. It will be posted in the restaurant, or ask for a brochure. Once you know how many calories are in the foods you normally eat, and practice counting, you will soon be able to look at a plate of food and "see" the number of calories on it. The following is a list of some common foods and their calories:

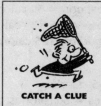

CATCH A CLUE

What Is a Calorie?

A calorie is a unit of measurement which defines how much energy a food provides. For instance, an apple provides eighty calories of energy.

Fast Food:
Burger King Whopper: 640 calories
McDonald's Big Mac: 562 calories
Wendy's French fries: 306 calories
Dairy Queen ice-cream cone: 190 calories

Prepared Meals:
Lasagna with meat: 1 piece = 398 calories
Macaroni with cheese: 1 cup = 230 calories
Hot dog and bun: 260 calories
Cheese pizza: 1 small piece = 290 calories

Dairy Products:
Skim milk: 1 cup = 86 calories
2% milk: 1 cup = 121 calories
Cheddar cheese: 1-inch cube = 114 calories
Ice cream, vanilla: 1 cup = 349 calories
Frozen yogurt, vanilla: 1 cup = 110 calories

Fats and Oils:
Butter: 1 tablespoon = 100 calories
Margarine: 1 tablespoon = 50 calories
Canola oil: 1 tablespoon = 125 calories
Olive oil: 1 tablespoon = 125 calories

Breads:
Bread: 1 slice = 65 calories
Crackers: 4 Saltines = 50 calories
Bagel: 1 small = 180 calories

Snacks:
Potato chips: 14 chips = 148 calories
Doughnut: 1 yeast = 235 calories
Graham crackers: 2 crackers = 60 calories
Tortilla chips: 1 ounce = 139 calories

The Count Begins

Don't get scared when you read the next sentence. One pound of body fat contains 3,500 calories. I know that sounds like a lot, but it's important information to know. If your goal is to lose one pound, you have to take in 3,500 calories less than you expend. If you want to lose ten pounds, you have to take in 35,000 calories less than you expend! OK, before you throw in the towel, remember that it's done over a lengthy span of time. You don't have to starve yourself by cutting out that many calories in a day or

Bagels Beware!

Watch out for the bagels at specialty bagel shops. One cinnamon-raisin bagel packs a whopping 300 calories! Add cream cheese on top, and it kicks up the calorie count to 400–500, depending on if you slather it on thick!

wow!

two. On the average, a deficit of 500 calories a day will bring about a one-pound weight loss in a week. But watch out! Just the opposite is true. Eating an excess of 500 calories a day for a week will bring about a one-pound weight gain at the end of that week! So counting calories will help you keep track of which end of the scales you're tipping.

DAILY CALORIC REQUIREMENTS

By knowing how many calories it takes to maintain your specific body weight, you can then set goals for altering your calorie consumption and ultimately losing weight. To figure this estimate, use the following equation:

Calorie Requirement:
body weight in pounds x 20

Example:

125 pounds x 20 = 2,500 calories a day.

So if it takes 2,500 calories to maintain 125 pounds, try dropping 500 calories a day to lose a pound a week. Or you could choose to walk for a half hour a day which would burn 150 calories, and then you would only need to eat 350 calories less a day.

Holy Cow!

One pound of body fat contains 3,500 calories!

wow!

CALORIES BURNED ON VARIOUS ACTIVITIES

Let's face it—we're not trying to gain weight. If you're anything like me, you are counting the calories you eat to know how many calories you have to burn in order to maintain or lose weight. Since many of us are sedentary most of the day, we're not burning many calories sitting at a desk or dusting the furniture. (Those of you who have jobs as bicycle couriers or postal carriers, you can skip this section.) Exercising will help burn a few more calories. Here is a list of activities and calories burned. This will show you how long you need to work out to burn off that cookie you had for dessert.

Walking: 3 mph = 5 cal/min
Running: 9-minute mile = 11.4 cal/min
Biking: 13 mph = 10 cal/min
Aerobic dance: medium intensity = 6.1 cal/min
Tennis: 6.4 cal/min

Setting Goals

When setting goals to count calories and lose weight, there are a few guidelines that will improve your chances of success.

1. Make a calorie logbook. Create a place where you can record what you eat (the foods and the amount of calories in each food) every day. Seeing it on paper makes it real and easier to see where you can shave off extra calories.

2. Be patient. Counting all those calories takes time. But you will get the hang of it, and after a while, you won't need to constantly be looking up each food for its calorie count.

wow!

Top Ten Goal Breakers:

10. Shopping while hungry
9. Valentine's Day chocoholic party
8. A long car trip with lots o' snacks
7. Date night at the movies with all the fixin's
6. A woe-is-me party after a breakup
5. Celebrating anything with dessert
4. Leftover Halloween candy
3. A dessert baking class
2. Christmas cookie trade
1. Thanksgiving Day dinner

3. Set attainable goals. Don't be overaggressive in cutting calories. It's easy to be gung-ho at the beginning and practically starve yourself, but resist the temptation. A healthy goal is to lose one to two pounds a week. Trying to eat less than the amount to do this is too restrictive, and you'll likely end up reverting back to old eating habits.

4. Plan for parties and special events. If you know you'll be going to an event where there will be a lot of high-fat and caloric foods, try not to eat as much during the rest of the day. This will allow more calories to spare to enjoy the special food. A better idea is to eat right before you go to the party so you won't be hungry and apt to eat those high-calorie foods.

5. Don't give up if you mess up. No one eats perfectly all the time. And there will be days when you'll go over your calorie limit, sometimes by a lot. But don't quit. Losing weight takes a consistent effort and a few extra calories here and there won't hurt.

6. Don't always skip dessert. It's OK to have a little something sweet if you're eating a healthy diet. Just be careful not to go overboard. Eating a small dessert will keep you from feeling deprived.

Being Aware of Calories

If you are serious about losing weight, take note of some common ways to become more aware of calories:

1. Frequently browse a list of foods and their caloric content to familiarize yourself with those you eat most often.
2. Keep that calorie list with you to help you make wise choices when faced with limited food options, for instance, eating out or while on the road.
3. Think before you eat. Always consider the implications of what you are eating. Ask yourself, *Will I be able to restrict myself more at the next meal because of what I'm eating now?*

DOWNSIDE OF BEING TOO AWARE

Sometimes people become so obsessed with counting calories that it begins to overwhelm their mental energies. Manipulating their diet to eat whatever they want becomes their focus and hobby. Either they can't enjoy anything sweet because of the guilt it causes, or they cut out healthy foods in order to eat junk food. Eventually they give up because they can't take the restrictions they've placed on themselves, or they get sick from the unhealthy foods they've consumed.

FRESH PERSPECTIVE

Food is meant for our nourishment. Its purpose is to keep us alive and give us energy. Ask God daily to help you keep food in perspective and to eat only what you need.

IS COUNTING CALORIES FOR YOU?

Counting calories takes some work and commitment, but after you get the hang of it, it'll become a natural part of your eating habits. You'll be surprised to find that when you try to eat the recommended number of servings of food from each of the food groups, you will have little appetite left for those high-calorie junk foods.

A Low-Fat Approach

Since fat has gotten such a bad rap, it's hard to believe that it actually has some redeeming qualities. With all the hype about it giving us double chins and thunder thighs, you'll be surprised to find that fat's main role in our bodies is to provide energy. Since it's pretty important to have a constant energy supply to keep our systems functioning, God created fat as a built-in reserve to protect us from ever being deprived of energy. Here's how it works: When your body has used up the energy it obtained from your most recent meal and whatever was stored in your muscles, your body begins to rely on its fat stores for energy. Unfortunately, our brain and heart need the energy provided by carbohydrates rather than that of fat, so at some point we have to eat or we will die. Bummer, I know.

Fat Is Fat, Right?

Nope. Just like there are different kinds of calories, there are different kinds of fat. Saturated, polyunsaturated, and monounsaturated. OK, now we're starting to sound technical. So as not to make this a confusing lesson in chemistry, let it be said that saturated fat is the unhealthiest kind of fat, followed by polyunsaturated and then monounsaturated fats. To help you tell the difference, remember that saturated fat is hard at room temperature while polyunsaturated fats are softer and melt easier. Generally speaking, animal fats are more saturated, while vegetable and fish oils are rich in polyunsaturated. Of the three meats, chicken fat is the least saturated while beef fat is the most saturated. (That is one reason why you should eat chicken rather than beef.) But what about olive oil and canola oil? Of all the fats, they are the best for you, because they are the highest in monounsaturated fats. But don't get carried away! They are still fat and very high in calories.

It's So Unfair

wow!

Remember our friend the polar bear who has ripples of fat under his thick fur coat? While he's sleeping the winter away, his body is metabolizing all that fat for energy to maintain his body temperature and other life processes. Come spring, he's a hundred or more pounds lighter than when he went to sleep. Wouldn't that be incredible if we could sleep off our fat like the polar bear?!

A Word About Hydrogenation

You might have heard about hydrogenated fat and wondered how that fits into the overall selection of fats. For those of you who remember back to your chemistry days, hydrogenation is a process where hydrogen molecules are added to the polyunsaturated fat molecules in a food to make it more solid. For example, without hydrogenation, margarine made of vegetable oils would not be solid at room temperature. So they add some hydrogen molecules to the open bonds in the oils which makes the margarine more solid and easier to work with. What a great idea, right? Unfortunately, hydrogenation makes a food less healthy. But how could adding hydrogen to something make it less healthy? Because hydrogenation diminishes a food's polyunsaturated content and makes it more saturated.

The Difference Between Cholesterol and Fat

People have gotten cholesterol confused with fat because cholesterol is found only in animal foods, which are the major sources of saturated fats, but cholesterol and fat are actually two different things. Everything you've heard about cholesterol is bad, right? Well, believe it or not, just like fat, cholesterol does have some redeeming qualities. More than nine-tenths

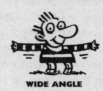

Fat Is Not All Bad

Fat serves many roles in the body.
1. Provides energy
2. Insulates the body from extreme temperatures
3. Protects internal organs
4. Maintains the structure and health of all cells

WIDE ANGLE

of the body's cholesterol is used to give cells their structure, plus it can be transformed into things like hormones, bile, and vitamin D. But cholesterol's one negative influence on the body has gotten all the bad press and for good reason. On its way into the cells from the bloodstream, some cholesterol is deposited on the artery walls. And it's this depositing of cholesterol in arteries that creates conditions ripe for heart attacks and strokes. So it's wise to limit animal products such as meats and eggs because they contain higher amounts of fat and cholesterol than other foods.

FAT IN FOODS

When you decide to take the low-fat approach to dieting, you need to be aware of where fat resides. It's pretty obvious in some cases, such as butter, margarine, and oils, but sometimes fat is invisible, and you need to be on the lookout. Here is a list of common foods with invisible fat:

- *Avocados, olives, nuts, and bacon.* These are essentially pure fat. An eighth of an avocado, a slice of bacon, or a little handful of peanuts can contain as much fat as a pat of butter!
- *Fried foods.* Anything fried is abundant in fat: potato chips, French fries, chicken fingers or nuggets, and fried chicken or fish.
- *Baked goods.* Pie crusts, pastries, doughnuts, sweet rolls, cookies, cakes, and biscuits. Watch out when you buy prepared baked goods at the grocery store. They will be loaded with fat.
- *Salad bars.* So many people think they are eating a low-fat/calorie diet when they choose the salad bar, but abundant fat is lurking there. It is simple to fill a plate with fifty percent of its calories coming from fat without even trying! Salad dressings, potato salad, macaroni salad, coleslaw, and even marinated beans are largely fat or oil.

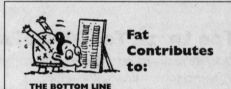

Fat Contributes to:

THE BOTTOM LINE

1. Obesity
2. Atherosclerosis (hardening of the arteries)
3. Diabetes
4. Cancer
5. Hypertension

- *Chocolate bars.* They actually contain more fat than they do sugar.
- *Creamy soups*. Even cream of mushroom soup prepared with water has sixty-six percent of its calories from fat.

The bottom line? Be on the lookout for fat.

Cholesterol in Foods

Cholesterol is found in animal foods. The following is a list of foods containing cholesterol:

1. Organ meat, such as liver and kidneys
2. Eggs—all the cholesterol is in the yolk
3. Shrimp
4. Veal
5. Chicken
6. Pork
7. Beef
8. Cheeses

TOO LITTLE, TOO MUCH FAT

Well, we're finally getting down to what everyone wants to know the most—how much fat can I eat every day? For the most part, society has sent the message that the less fat you eat and the less body fat you have, the healthier you are. But that is not necessarily the case. Like we said before, fat is actually benefi-cial, and it is harmful to ingest too much or too little of it. Unfortunately, in our country it's much easier to ingest too much of it.

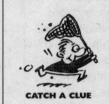

CATCH A CLUE

Recommended Daily Fat Intake:

Thirty percent of your day's total calories

HOW MUCH FAT?

It's time to talk about the nitty-gritty details of exactly how much fat we should be eating a day. The guidelines recommend that total fat intake should not exceed thirty percent of your day's total calories. Just stay calm—I know it doesn't sound like a lot, but let's figure out how much that is for you in particular. First, you have to know your daily calorie requirement.

Daily Calorie Requirement:
Body weight x 20
Example: 125 pounds x 20 = 2500 calories

Now to find out your daily fat requirement use the following equations:
Fat Requirement in Calories:
calorie requirement x percent fat recommended
Example: 2500 calories x 30 percent = 750 calories

To translate fat calories into grams of fat:
Fat Requirement in Grams:
Grams of fat = number of calories divided by 9
Example: 750 calories divided by 9 = 83 grams of fat

It is easier to keep track of how many fat grams you eat a day. So once you know the number of fat grams you should be eating to stay within thirty percent of your caloric need, you can easily monitor how many grams of fat are going into your mouth.

FAT WATCH

You've heard it a million times, but we wanted to say it again—fast food is very high in fat. But just how high? A McDonald's Big Mac and French fries pack in about forty-five grams of fat. So if your fat requirement is sixty-two grams, then you've just eaten almost all of your daily requirement in one meal! So when making a fast-food pit stop, be on the lookout for fat and choose wisely—a grilled chicken sandwich and hold the fries.

LOW-FAT CHOICES

Here are some ways to limit the fat and cholesterol in your diet.
Choose:
• vegetables and fruits, cereals and beans
• fish, and poultry without skin
• nonfat milk
• lean meats

Limit:
• oils
• fats
• egg yolks
• fried foods
• baked goods

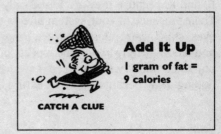

Add It Up
1 gram of fat =
9 calories

CATCH A CLUE

Fat-Free Food Frenzy

With the creation of "fat-free" foods, some people thought they had died and gone to hog heaven. Where else can you eat ice cream, cookies, and chips that actually taste good without any fat?! But there is a downside. "Fat-free" foods *are not* calorie

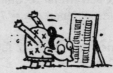

THE BOTTOM LINE

Downsides to Fat-Free Foods

1. High in calories
2. Low nutrient value
3. Feelings of hunger soon after eating

free. We repeat. "Fat-free" foods *are not* calorie free. Many of these foods still have just as many calories as their fat-filled counterparts. And remember, calories add up to pounds. The fat-free sweets have a lot of sugar, while foods such as chips are extremely high in salt to make them more palatable. The downside to fat-free foods is that because they don't have any fat, your feeling of "fullness" doesn't last very long, so you'll get hungry again soon. Ever noticed how after eating a high-fat meal such as fried chicken and mashed potatoes with gravy, you're not hungry again for a long time? It's because fat takes longer to digest. So if you eat a meal that contains no fat, it won't be long before you're raiding the candy machine for a snack.

CONS TO LOW-FAT EATING

While eating a low-fat diet is the healthiest way to eat, there are some dangers associated with a low, low-fat diet. To some people, if low fat is good, then no fat is better, and they restrict their diet to an extremely low level of fat. But a no-fat diet does not mean a healthier diet. In fact, if you are not eating fat, you are at risk for not getting the vitamins A, D, E, and K, because they are found only in the fat and oily parts of food. Their presence in your system affects the health and function of your eyes, skin, gastrointestinal tract, lungs, bones, teeth, nervous system, and blood—pretty important aspects of your body, I'd say! It just doesn't pay to be thin if you can't see, have lost your teeth, and your skin is flaking away because you quit eating fat.

Pros to Low-Fat Eating

The number one pro for eating a low-fat diet is that you will lose weight. By taking in less fat, you automatically will be taking in less calories, thus weight loss is inevitable. But eating a low-fat diet also has health benefits. Eating a high-fat diet aggravates the risk of hypertension, diabetes, cancer, and atherosclerosis (hardening of the arteries), which increases your chance of suffering a heart attack or stroke. So the pros of eating a low-fat diet are basically the difference between life and death. Not only will you be living longer, this type of diet will help

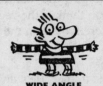

WIDE ANGLE

I Was Such a Flake

"I was on a kick once where I thought I could lose weight by not eating any fat. I limited my diet to things like dry cereal, carrot sticks, fruit, rice cakes, and cooked, dry pasta. After a while I began to notice that my skin was flaky, I looked pale, and my hair dried out. I felt lethargic and gross most of the day. It wasn't until a routine physical when the doctor noticed and shared with me the health risks of what I was doing that I changed my eating habits."
—Lynn, Sedona, Arizona

preserve your health as you age. And who wouldn't want to be able to play with their grandkids and enjoy life when they're eighty, ninety, or even a hundred years old?!

Is the Low-Fat Diet for You?

It's true that fat helps make foods taste delicious, but the consequence of excessive fats to your health can be severe. Most people picture low-fat eating as bland and boring, but

DON'T FORGET

Low-Fat Diet Pros:

1. Weight loss
2. Disease prevention
3. Health preservation

eating healthy does not mean you have to eat without pleasure. Here are some common ways to make the low-fat diet work for you:

1. Use fat only where you'll notice its taste benefits.
2. Substitute other foods for fat when you won't notice.
3. Use fat substitutes where you can.
4. Learn to enjoy foods with less fat in or on them. (It really is possible!)

And remember: Fat has its place in your diet; just be careful not to exceed your needs.

Vegetarians

Below we're going to give you four descriptions. We'd like you to pick the person whom you think is the vegetarian and put a mark in that box. Then put a different mark in the box of the person whom you think is not a vegetarian.

❐ Bill is an athletic trainer. He's divorced and lives by himself in a small two-bedroom apartment. He usually eats on the run and doesn't always eat right.

❐ Lila is a gardener. While her husband goes off to work, Lila spends her day tending to her plants in the greenhouse behind their house.

❐ Steve is an activist. He doesn't hold down a regular job but makes his living picking up odd jobs wherever he can find them. He believes people should live off the earth and that animals are treated cruelly.

❐ Sally is a housewife who runs a growing home-based business. Both her children are in school, and her husband works outside the home.

Finished? Great. Ready for the answer?

They're all vegetarians.

Vegetarians are often seen as people who are militant about animal rights or the environment. And they're easily pigeonholed into being thought of as people who deserve to be marginalized and left outside society.

These days, though, being a vegetarian is becoming more respected. Vegetarians are more difficult to pick out of a crowd. Before, they were largely misunderstood. These days, their diet has been made popular through movie star endorsements of the diet and an abundance of promotion about the vegetarian lifestyle.

PROFILE: THE VEGETARIAN

What is a vegetarian? It's simple, really. A vegetarian is someone who's decided to eat only vegetables as his source of food. Now, within that classification lie several different categories of vegetarians based on what foods they eat. Here's a simple breakdown:

• *Vegans*—the most dedicated vegetarians, they eat exclusively plant products, and no meat, dairy, or fish products at all.

- *Lactovegetarians*—also eat dairy products, but not eggs, meat, or fish.
- *Ovolactovegetarians*—include both eggs and dairy products in the menu, but no meat or fish.
- *Fruitarians*—eat only raw fruit and supplement with vegetables.

Even within this framework, there are hundreds of differing philosophies and diets. And reasons for being a vegetarian differ as much as the diets do. For example, some vegetarians choose the diet for health reasons. Others choose to be vegetarians to make a stand against animal cruelty.

HEALTH OR PHILOSOPHY?

Many people choose to become vegetarians due to the increased risks involved in eating meat. However, several other reasons exist for becoming a vegetarian.

- **Philosophical:** Some people have a basic problem with eating meat. They're against killing any animal. They believe that humans weren't created to consume other living things.
- **Theoretical:** Some studies indicate that the human intestines are too long and are not intended to digest meat. Animals that are obviously intended to eat meat (those with longer, sharper teeth) have shorter intestines perfect for digesting meat.
- **Sociological:** Some people feel that animals prepared for human consumption are treated poorly. As a result, they oppose the preparation of meat for consumption.
- **Medical:** Some health technicians have ample data to suggest that meat harms the human body. Some claim that it's prepared in an unsafe way. Others feel that chemicals in meat harm us.

FOUR NEW FOOD GROUPS

Vegetarians have reinvented the four basic food groups to fit their diet. Here's a snapshot of the four vegetarian food groups.

Vegetables: Dark green vegetables like broccoli, kale, and collards
Whole Grains: Bread, rice, pasta, and tortillas
Fruit: Those high in vitamin C, like citrus fruits and strawberries
Legumes: Also known as beans, peas, and lentils

FOOD YOU CAN EAT

What's the most daunting task you might face trying the vegetarian diet? Yep—food. You might feel like you're entering a lifestyle that offers you nothing to eat, while stigmatizing you as some wacko who has some problem with meat.

The truth is, you don't give up too much when you decide to go vegetarian. The American Dietetic Association suggests that you:

• Choose a variety of foods, including whole grains, vegetables, fruits, legumes, nuts, seeds, dairy products, and eggs.

• Choose whole, unrefined foods and minimize your intake of highly sweetened, fatty, and heavily refined foods.

• Choose a variety of fruits and vegetables.

• If you choose to eat animal and dairy foods, choose those that are lower in fat.

The Pros and Cons of Being a Vegetarian

ADVANTAGES

Losing Weight

If you're into this diet thing to lose weight, chances are with this diet, you'll succeed. That's due to a variety of factors. You're changing the food that your body takes in, you're removing some major fat content, and you're eating food that is used more efficiently by your body. And because your body is using the food you're eating more efficiently, you just might be able to eat more.

You've Got the Answer

Everyone has their reasons. If you're considering this diet, you probably have some of your own. In the space provided, write your reasons for choosing this diet.

WIDE ANGLE

_____

_____

_____

_____

Cholesterol

When you remove meat, you remove another way your body takes in cholesterol. Now, this isn't to say that your cholesterol level will go through the basement, but it just might get significantly lower. To check this out, consider getting your cholesterol checked before you try out this diet, then get it checked again after you've been on it a while. You just might see a difference.

Being Sick Less

Meat is treated with a lot of things like hormones and chemicals. The result? Well, sometimes those chemicals can make people sick. Now, not *real* sick, but sometimes kind of sick. So when you remove meat from your diet, you remove another chance for something to make you sick. There is one drawback to being sick less though. If you're sick less often, you'll be at work more.

DISADVANTAGES

As with any diet, you'll experience some disadvantages. Here are some.

Missing B_{12}

B_{12} isn't a fighter plane. It's a vital chemical that your body need for things like memory retention, stress management, and your attention span.

When you choose the vegetarian diet, you give up foods that supply you with this vitamin. Care must be taken to replace this chemical by supplementing your diet with vitamins.

Eating Out

The first thing you'll notice is that your choices at restaurants are limited. Most eateries don't cater specifically to vegetarians. How do you conquer this? Simple. Get comfortable with what you're doing. Before you go out, read up on foods you can eat. Spend time cooking for yourself *before* you go out to eat.

Embarrassment

It's not *really* a health consideration, but remember this: When you go out to eat with friends who knew you as a meat eater, you might get questioned about your change in eating habits. Be prepared to explain yourself when hanging out with friends. Spend time writing out your beliefs about what you're doing. It might be a simple explanation like, "I just want to eat healthier." Or you might want to go into brief detail about some philosophical or religious beliefs. Just be prepared to be questioned.

Take It a Step Further

CATCH A CLUE

If you want to try this diet, but aren't sure that it's totally for you, consider trying it out for a day or two. If you like what's happening to your body, extend your experiment. If you're unsure, it's okay to end it.

Lack of Protein?

Launching into this diet requires some caution. You're changing what you put into your body. More specifically, you're removing meat—but that doesn't mean that you're giving up protein. Beans, for example, replace some of the protein that you won't be getting without meat.

Finding Foods

One disadvantage (which we'll talk more about later) is that your food becomes more difficult to find. Before you began this diet, you probably were able to eat whatever you got your hands on. Now, though, you can't just eat anywhere you want or anything you want. Even buying your food becomes more difficult—not all grocery stores carry vegetarian foods.

Shopping Options

If you've decided to begin the vegetarian diet and if you've begun looking for food, you'll notice that there's not a whole lot available to you. Where should you buy your food?

Well, if you're looking for meals prepared according to your specific diet, try the following three options:

Large Chains: If you live in or near a large city, you'll probably be able to find large grocery stores that offer vegetarian meals. If they don't offer them, or if you live in a small city, look for foods that you'll be able to prepare at home according to your diet.

Natural Food Stores: Most natural food stores offer vegetarian foods or even dedicate aisles to the vegetarian diet.

Vegetarian Food Stores: Check out the Yellow Pages to see if there's a vegetarian food store in your city. Some larger cities offer entire stores that are dedicated to providing foods specifically for vegetarians.

Food-Finding Options: If those three ideas don't help you out for where you live, try these options:

Surf the Internet for on-line grocery stores. There are a lot of grocery businesses that offer on-line ordering and convenient shipping. To find them just do a search with your favorite search engine. Search for keywords like "Vegetarian Foods," "On-line Groceries," and "Stores on the Net."

Look for a support group. We're not saying that if you're a vegetarian, then you need a support group. But if you're having difficulty finding vegetarian foods in your city, then others have had the same problem. Ask around to see if there are groups of people in your city who meet to exchange vegetarian recipes or offer ideas for finding great places to buy food.

Surviving as a Vegetarian

Deciding to make the change to vegetarianism is easier than actually following through with your decision. As with any diet, you'll encounter things that try and knock you off track.

FIRST THREE MONTHS

We want to be totally honest with you. Trying this diet is not easy, and it's not for everyone. In the first three months you'll be confronted with several harsh realities. Your body will try and get adjusted—which means there might be times you crave meat. If you do give in, don't feel discouraged. One phrase might help you stay focused. Here it is: Keep going!

Famous Vegetarians

Some famous people have worn (or wear) the vegetarian tag: Drew Barrymore, Thomas Edison, Chelsea Clinton, Brad Pitt, Weird Al Yankovic, and Sir Isaac Newton.

WOW!

KEEP GOING!

When you feel a craving to give up, or you're not sure you've made the right decision, commit yourself to stay on track. After the first three months, if you're still not satisfied, consider switching. But not until then.

Set a Goal

We want to encourage you to set your goal for being a vegetarian, because being a vegetarian can be much more than just a diet. It can be a lifestyle. So, what do you want to accomplish with your new lifestyle? Just get healthy? Send a message to people you meet? Help conserve living things?

Whatever your reasoning behind being a vegetarian, be sure to phrase what you want to accomplish in a sentence. If you want to just get healthy, you might want to say something like, "I want to be living a

"Quit Buggin' Me"

If you feel you'll have a tough time explaining your philosophy or new eating habits, consider what one person does.

WOW!

"I just state that I don't eat things that have eyes and might want to run away from me. If that doesn't work, I say, 'I don't eat DEAD animals.' I am never bothered about my vegetarianism again, it seems."

**(Quote from
http://vegetarian.about.com/library/weekly/m
current.htm?pid=2757&cob=home)**

healthier lifestyle in six months." If you're trying to raise consciousness, try and phrase that in a readable and easily memorable sentence. Then, at the beginning of your day, repeat that statement to yourself several times to help you to focus and encourage yourself.

Think for a moment. What's your goal? Can you phrase it into something you can remember? Write out your ideas here.

• _____

• _____

• _____

Are YOU a Vegetarian?

Before you leap into the world of vegetarianism, ask yourself the following questions:
• Is meat an essential part of my daily diet? Can I survive without it?
• Am I offended by the way they process meat?
• Am I concerned about the effects meat has on my body?

If, after answering these questions, you feel God leading you to pursue a vegetarian diet, bravo! Happy eating!

Sugar Free

THE BASIC IDEA

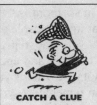

CATCH A CLUE

Men vs. Women

You know how it is with diets. Men lose weight so much more quickly than women. *SUGAR BUSTERS!* authors note that women often have a greater success with this plan. You go, girls!

1. Certain foods (meaning sugars and those starches which quickly convert to sugars in your body) stimulate your pancreas to create the hormone insulin.
2. Insulin functions in your body by controlling the sugar in your blood on the high end. If the sugar gets too high, the insulin starts shuffling it into cells for storage. This means you gain weight.
3. Therefore, if you cut out the foods that stimulate the insulin (sugars and starches which quickly convert to sugars) then the insulin won't kick in so much and you won't gain as much weight.
4. In fact, what will kick in is the hormone glucagon which keeps your blood sugar level from getting too low by using up the substance that the insulin has already stored in your cells.

Great system, huh? According to the authors of *SUGAR BUSTERS!* no one has really made the insulin/fat connection known before. Doctors who have specialized in diabetes have long known that once they up a patient's insulin his or her weight increases, but the issue they were studying was not weight loss, but diabetes, so no one made the connection. . .at least no one that was listened to. . .until recently.

The best-selling book *SUGAR BUSTERS!* was written by three doctors and one corporate CEO. The authors are quick to point out that low-fat diets and foods have not worked. Why? Because in order to take fats out of food, food manufacturers have added sugar in one form or another. As the general population has eaten more and more of these fat-free foods, they have put more and more sugar into their bodies and, in truth, either not lost weight or regained the weight they lost.

The authors of *SUGAR BUSTERS!* further declare that some of us have even become "insulin resistant" which means we have taken in so much sugar that our bodies are now resistant to insulin. The end result is that our body has to create much more insulin to keep our sugar levels in check. This overworks our pancreas and contributes to other health issues.

DON'T COUNT CALORIES

What???? You don't count calories? Then how can this diet work? Well, you don't count calories—you count how fast a food turns into sugar. *SUGAR BUSTERS!* calls this the Glycemic Index. You'll have to buy the book to find out exactly what a Glycemic Index looks like, but basically it will show you which foods turn immediately to sugar and, according to the authors, right to fat. Even though some of these foods will coincide with the high-calorie foods that you've always stayed away from, you'll find some surprises among the foods on the list. It can also be refreshing to evaluate your food by a new measure. Counting calories gets soooo old once you've done it ten or twenty years. Here's a new way to look at food.

The Plan

So the plan is first to stay away from the obvious sugars, like candy bars, cookies, cakes, sugar-sweetened colas, and ice cream. Then the plan is to stay away from the not-so-obvious sugars, such as white bread, white potatoes, white rice, corn, and carrots. To make their point, the authors of *SUGAR BUSTERS!* ask you to take a potato skin with the potato inside scooped out, fill the potato skin with white sugar and then ask yourself, "Would I eat that?" Their premise is that is exactly what you are eating when you eat a simple

Yay or Nay?

Do's

Green beans
Sweet potatoes
Grapefruit
DON'T FORGET Tomatoes
Certain fruits, but by themselves, not with other foods

Don'ts

White bread
Pasta
Refined grains
Carrots
Bananas

starch like a potato that changes immediately into sugar in your body.

You should replace these high-glycemic foods with more whole grain, unrefined foods such as lean meats, fiber-rich starches and veggies, and natural and unrefined sugars such as whole fruits (see the good and bad fruit lists in this chapter).

SUGAR BUSTERS! also gives you info about how to combine your foods, for instance, not combining fruit with other foods but eating fruit alone.

WIDE ANGLE

Interesting Tidbits

Fruits should be eaten alone because they digest more quickly that way.

The reason red wine is better for you (in terms of the Glycemic Index) is because the grape skins are involved in the making of red wine. Those skins contain Vitamin P which helps your blood in ways that are right up the *SUGAR BUSTERS!'* alley. If you don't want to drink red wine on this diet, though, you can take an aspirin a day and eat white or red grapes, skin and all.

Multiple, smaller meals throughout the day are better than two or three big ones.

Appropriate portion sizes should fit nicely on a dinner plate, not running over, and no seconds or thirds.

Don't eat right before you go to bed.

Don't wash down your food: It keeps you from chewing well and dilutes the stomach's digestive juices.

There's plenty more where these tips came from. If you're interested, check out *SUGAR BUSTERS!*

SUGAR BUSTERS! claims to be able to reconnect you with those foods that you have given up for years in your unsuccessful attempts to lose weight and still enable you to lose those extra pounds.

WHAT THE CRITICS SAY

Many critics say that the basic premise of this program is not so different from Dr. Atkins's diet (which most people refer to as a high-protein diet). Dr. Atkins even cites the dangers of insulin in his research. So where is the new information? Perhaps this isn't a new diet so much as a new spin on a standard diet highlighting the same enemy (sugar) in a new way.

Also, for any diet that cuts out one type of food

THE BOTTOM LINE

Secret Weapon

SUGAR BUSTERS! claims to help improve your chances against these contributing factors to arterial disease:
- **High blood pressure**
- **Diabetes**
- **Elevated cholesterol**
- **Elevated triglycerides**
- **Obesity**
- **Stress**
- **High blood sugar**

completely, there are ten critics who say that in the end it's not the healthiest way to go. Often, they say that a drastic decrease in carbs will create a more dramatic craving for sugars. They also point out that when it's carbohydrates being cut, often the fats rise to make up the difference and you are back in a cardiovascular predicament.

The final word from critics seems to be that any food in excess will be converted to fat. This diet makes the carbohydrates out to be the only foods that do so. They claim that it's not the insulin that causes the weight; it's the weight that causes the insulin. If so, then this diet has no benefit over a balanced diet and may have some harmful risks.

Diet Fads

A Look at Some Memorable Diets

Hit diets, just like hit songs, tend to have a hook. They have one unique drum that they beat loudly to draw attention. Whether it's sugars or carbohydrates or calories or body types or. . .whatever, diets have to have a hook to draw any attention to themselves or to make any money (if they're a book or a clinic). While diets today tout the insulin level and certain food groups, there really hasn't been any groundbreaking change in the way that diets work. After you've read through the hook and the hype, most diets will tell you to eat in moderation, to drink plenty of water, to exercise, and (for most) to eat more small meals rather than a few big ones.

The function of diets tends to be not new information, but the distraction from the doldrums of doing the right thing day after day. If we are distracted by counting glycemic indexes or grams of something, then we get through more days without noticing that we've been doing the right thing for several days running. We get distracted with this new system of eating and living and, until it gets old, we might do some good for ourselves.

Diet fads come and go. They are spread through the Internet, word of mouth (like we said, the Internet) and even official sources like institutions. Often the more outrageous the hook of the diet the more attention it gets at first. Some of them are bizarre. Some of them have worked. Some have stayed the course. Some of them have changed people's lives. Here are a few you might have passed on your journey.

THE BANANA, WEENIE, AND EGG

Remember this? There were several variations. The most memorable was to eat nine bananas the first day (Breakfast = 3, Lunch = 3, Dinner = 3). The second day you ate nine weenies divided into three meals. The third day you ate nine boiled eggs the same way. On the fourth day you ate three bananas for breakfast, three weenies for lunch, and three boiled eggs for dinner. Did you lose weight? The mystery diet wizards who concocted this diet said you'd lose ten pounds. If we could find someone who had ever finished the diet, we would know if it worked!

THE MAYO CLINIC DIET

You usually receive this diet from a friend. It's usually a copy of a copy of a copy of a copy (ad infinitum) of a typewritten sheet. This sheet will tell you that this diet is used in the cardiovascular department at the Mayo Clinic. The sheet will tell you that you can stay on the diet for as long as you need to.

The Mayo Clinic Diet is really a form of the famous Atkins's Diet Revolution. You are required to forego starches and sugars and fill up on proteins and veggies. In fact, the diet tells you that the more you eat the more you'll lose, so you should eat until you can't hold anymore. (Compulsive eaters, rejoice!)

For twelve days you drink grapefruit juice with each meal, eat bacon and eggs (no toast) for breakfast, and meat and salad or green beans for lunch and supper. For an evening snack you can have milk or tomato juice. After the first three days the weight starts dropping and every twelve days you take two days off and start all over.

Usually this diet leads to a very high fat intake and an altering of some bodily functions, but it guarantees ten pounds in ten days, and for some, it delivers.

CABBAGE SOUP DIET

The hook for this diet is a recipe for a cabbage-based soup. You can eat as much of the soup as you want and you'll feel full, but be prepared. . . some flatulence could occur. (You don't know what "flatulence" means? It means no one will stand downwind of you.)

With the soup you have a modest food plan. Eating the soup gets old. The food plan might work for you without the soup.

There are people who have lost weight on this diet. We just don't know if they can look at a cabbage again.

LIQUID SUPPLEMENTS

Optifast and Slimfast are probably the most famous of these kinds of weight loss plans. Due to a good marketing department and some honest successes, Slimfast is probably the most recognizable. Some people just drink the liquids and forego eating until they have lost the weight they want to lose. Others use the can or "shake" for one or two meals a day and then have regular food the rest of the time.

The drinks are convenient. There's no getting around that. They give you something to do for a meal that lowers your food choices to none. But when you look at the calories and the amount of healthy, good-tasting food that you could have for the same calories, you have to wonder why you're drinking the "shake" instead of eating the food. Of course if you could eat only that many calories for a meal you wouldn't be buying the shake in the first place.

What's Out There Today

DIET CENTERS AND SELF-HELP PROGRAMS

Each of these programs except Overeaters Anonymous works with a low-calorie, lifestyle modification plan that works toward a one- to two-pound weight loss per week and a changed life.

Weight Watchers: They've been around from the beginning. They've changed with the times. They've updated with the research. They've raised their prices, but who hasn't? There's almost always a chapter within driving distance and they are waiting with a smile and a scale. If you haven't checked out Weight Watchers in years, you might want to look again.

Overeaters Anonymous: This is a twelve-step program based on the same principles as Alcoholics Anonymous. It isn't a group that is geared toward weight loss. It is a group that is geared toward a healthy relationship with food, yourself, and your higher power.

Diet Workshop: You can buy their food or not. You'll be expected to exercise and to lose one to two pounds a week. This is behavior modification all the way, working toward a lifestyle change.

TOPS (Take Off Pounds Sensibly): TOPS is all about accountability. You choose your plan and bring it into the group, then you help each other stay on that plan.

Jenny Craig: You are required to buy their prepackaged food at first. As you modify your behavior and lifestyle, you begin to plan your own menus and buy your own food.

CONTROLLED CARB DIETS

New Atkins Diet Revolution: High proteins and low carbs are the earmarks of this food plan. It was the first and still stands strong. Dr. Atkins tells us all that those starches are what keep us overweight. This was a controversial plan from the beginning, but it has stuck around.

Protein Power: Insulin is the culprit. Carbohydrates cause your body to produce insulin so you've got to cut back on them and make your body a weight-losing machine in the process. The critics have the same complaints with this diet as with others of its type.

Sugar Busters!: Once again, insulin stimulated by carbohydrates is the villain. Get rid of that sugar in its simple and complex forms and you can lose weight with the best of them.

The Zone: This diet is also called the 40-30-30 diet. It is based on hormones rather than calories. It's another version of the same story that started with Dr. Atkins in the seventies. Don't eat all carbs. They don't help as much as you think they do.

OTHER BEST-SELLERS

Eat Right 4 Your Type: Your food plan is based on your blood type. This is an unusual plan. No other research has reflected the conclusions of this author. In short, Type As tend toward vegetarianism. Type Bs tend toward red meat and fish. Type Os tend toward high protein and low carbs. Who knew?

New Beverly Hills Diet: The hook for this diet is in the combination of foods eaten. Fruit is a premium but never eaten with meat (reminiscent of *Sugar Busters!).* According to this plan, the combinations of food cause the enzymes in your body to help you lose weight.

Words of Warning and Wisdom

Beware of. . .

Diets that ignore a whole food group: At the bottom of it all, a balanced food plan is the best—all of the food groups in the right proportion. Most diets are based not so much on deleting a food group, but rather minimizing one or more. Don't depend on one kind of food to help you lose weight (that would be trusting a gimmick). It's the whole plan that will make the difference.

Diets that claim an easy, quick-fix weight loss without effort: You should know by now that there is no easy fix. You know the difference between water weight loss and the real thing. You know that the faster you lose the weight the easier it will be to put it back on. You know that weight loss is hard work. Don't lay your money down for anyone who tells you any different.

Diets that claim you can overeat and still lose weight: Don't let the "you can eat it all and lose weight" sermon make you believe that there is a shortcut. Haven't you heard? "It took you a long time to put it on; it will take you a long time to take it off." If this kind of diet catches you every time, then let that be your warning signal to dig deeper into why you eat. Is it fear? Is it anger? Is it boredom? Face the journey to discover your relationship with food, not just the weight you want to lose.

Avoiding the Weight Yo-Yo

LIFESTYLE

It's been said more times than you can count. You've probably said it yourself. It has to be a lifestyle. Many of the diet books that stock current shelves (perhaps your own) start out with the same sermon. You have to change your eating for life. You have to change the way you live.

One of the dangers with the more faddish, bizarre food plans is that you adopt a temporary way of eating, one that cannot be maintained for a lifetime, and then when you finish the diet, you are left in the same dilemma that you started out in. "How do I eat food, the right kinds, and the right proportions so that I am an appropriate weight for my height and body type?" If you haven't answered that question for yourself during the process of the diet, then there's a big challenge ahead for keeping that weight off.

EXERCISE

The jury really is not out on exercise. The jury is back and the judge has pronounced a sure and certain verdict, with the terms of the sentencing in permanent ink. There is no reprieve from any governor that will change the fact that exercise is one of the only sure and certain ways that you can keep from gaining back the weight you have lost on a diet.

Morning exercise in particular is valuable in this process. It sets your perspective first thing in the morning. It gets your metabolism working with you. It helps you make the right choices. If you want your weight off for life, start walking, or running, or biking, or stepping, or. . .

Our Own Approach

"I'm way too busy." "I don't have the time." "I'm sure I eat better than most." "I'm going to start a healthier lifestyle next month (or at the start of the New Year), when life will be more relaxed." Do you ever find yourself making excuses like these for why you should put off eating healthier? The options are as endless as the fast food restaurant choices that tempt our taste buds on a daily basis.

To summarize our suggestions so far, here are some basic guidelines to follow when eating healthy.

• Eat a variety of foods.
• Maintain a healthy weight.
• Choose a diet low in fat, saturated (hard) fat, and cholesterol.
• Choose a diet with plenty of vegetables, fruits, and grain products.
• Use sugars only in moderation.
• Use salt and sodium only in moderation.

UP CLOSE AND PERSONAL

To make these suggestions practical, we've devised a Healthy Eating Plan Sheet (pages 86–87) that can be personalized and stuck on your refrigerator door to serve as a reminder while you cook and snack. This plan sheet was created to follow the recommendations of the U.S. Department of Health and Human Services and the National Research Council of the Food and Nutrition Board. Their recommendations include the following:

• Energy: balance intake and expenditure of calories to maintain a desirable body weight.
• Fat: less than 20-30% of total calories should be from fat.
• Saturated fat: less than 10% of total calories should be from hard fat.
• Cholesterol: less than 300 mg per day.
• Sodium: 1.1–3.3 g/day.
• Fiber: 25–30 g/day.

YOUR IDEAL WEIGHT

You can figure out a rough estimate of your "desirable body weight" with the following rule of thumb. Women should weigh one hundred pounds for the first five feet of height, plus five pounds for each inch above five feet. Men should weigh 106 pounds for the first five feet, plus six pounds for each inch above five feet.

There are a couple of ways to figure out how many calories you need each day to maintain your desired weight. One method is to multiply the weight in pounds by eleven for women and twelve for men. So, for example, the desirable weight for a 5'3" woman would be 115 pounds (100+5+5+5), and her daily caloric needs would be 1265 calories (115 x 11).

You can figure out how much of your calories should be from the different food sources—fat, protein (meat and dairy), and carbohydrates (pretty much everything else)—by remembering the following: fat has nine calories in every gram, while protein and carbohydrates contain only four calories in every gram. So, for example, the 5'3" woman, who should get approximately 1300 calories each day with no more than thirty percent of these calories from fat, should try to eat less than forty-three grams of fat every day (1300 kcals multiplied by 0.30, then divided by 9 kcals/g). A healthy diet should have no more than twenty to thirty percent of its calories from fat, fifteen percent from protein, and sixty to seventy percent from carbohydrates.

Make the Healthy Eating Plan Sheet personal for yourself by remembering how many calories you need for your desired weight, and remembering how many calories should be from the different food sources. Using this as a guide, figure out how many different servings from the different groups you need. Eat the lowest number of servings if you are on the low end of calories needed (1600 or less), and the highest number of servings if you need more calories (2000 or more).

An important thing to know about this plan sheet is that some foods are included in more than one listing. Take cantaloupe for example. If you eat one fourth of a cantaloupe, you should cross off one serving of vitamin C foods and two servings of green leafy/yellow fruits and vegetables. Also, it is important to cross off fat servings when eating dairy products or meats.

To Sum Up

Being honest with yourself, you may not be someone who could follow a plan in so much detail. But take heart! Healthy eating can still be for you! Just remember some of the basic guidelines from this book, and follow these easy suggestions.

- **Pay attention to the new food labels.** They give information about the serving size and number of servings per container, plus information on calories, fat, and fiber. A simple rule of thumb is to avoid foods that contain more than ten to twenty-five percent of the daily value of things you are trying to avoid (i.e. fat, hard fat, or sodium).
- **Choose low-fat items whenever possible.** An easy way to cut out extra fat without too much of the flavor is to try some low-fat products out on the market today. This is especially great in the dairy department! Lean cuts of meat, poultry, and fish are also good choices.
- **Consider the Food Guide Pyramid.** The new Pyramid makes healthy eating recommendations easier to understand. Following the Pyramid will easily lower calories, fat, cholesterol, salt, and sugar, and increase vitamins, minerals, fiber, and other nutrients in your diet.
- **Avoid processed, packaged, and prepared foods containing added fat, salt, and sugar.** Processed foods are considered the major source of sodium and sugar in the American diet today.
- **Limit the use of salt and sugar in cooking and at the table.** This suggestion is mostly aimed at those who use a lot of these items. If you can't stand the thought of eating your food without these, try adding small amounts at the table, rather than adding them during cooking.

Just remember, you won't automatically start eating healthier, especially if you aren't motivated to change. It has to be a heart decision first. Also realize that mistakes are human and it doesn't help to beat yourself up over an occasional "slip." The point is to not feel like you are on a constant restricted "diet." You're trying to eat healthier for life. So an occasional indulgence can be good. . .as long as it's occasional!

Daily Servings

6 or more	**Whole Grains and Legumes**		
	1 slice whole grain bread (whole wheat, whole rye)	Sun	☐☐☐☐☐☐☐☐☐
	1/2 bagel, hamburger bun, English muffin	Mon	☐☐☐☐☐☐☐☐☐
	1/2 cup whole grain/high protein pasta	Tues	☐☐☐☐☐☐☐☐☐
	3-4 crackers	Wed	☐☐☐☐☐☐☐☐☐
	3/4-1 cup dry cereal, whole grain, no added sugar	Thurs	☐☐☐☐☐☐☐☐☐
	1/2 cup cooked brown or wild rice	Fri	☐☐☐☐☐☐☐☐☐
	2 t wheat germ (add to anything if not healthy)	Sat	☐☐☐☐☐☐☐☐☐
	1/2 cup cooked beans (navy, black, kidney) or peas		
	2"x2"x1" cornbread (nondegerminated meal)		

2-3 with:	**Protein**		
2 animal	3/4 cup lowfat cottage cheese	Sun	☐☐☐☐
1 nut, beans	1 3/4 cup lowfat yogurt	Mon	☐☐☐☐
	3 oz. Swiss, cheddar, lowfat cheese	Tues	☐☐☐☐
	2 large whole eggs	Wed	☐☐☐☐
	3 1/2 oz. tuna (packed in water), fish, or shrimp	Thurs	☐☐☐☐
	2 1/2 oz. white meat chicken/turkey	Fri	☐☐☐☐
	5 oz. clam, crab, lobster	Sat	☐☐☐☐
	3 oz. lean beef, pork, dark meat chicken		
	4 oz. fatty beef		
	Snacks: nuts and seeds, whole-grain baked goods, yogurt, hard cheese		

3 (800 + mg Ca)	**Calcium-Rich Foods**		
	8 oz. skim milk	Sun	☐☐☐☐
	1/2 cup evaporated skim milk	Mon	☐☐☐☐
	1 3/4 cups lowfat cottage cheese	Tues	☐☐☐☐
	1 1/2 oz. cheddar, American, Swiss cheese	Wed	☐☐☐☐
	1 cup lowfat/nonfat yogurt	Thurs	☐☐☐☐
	1/3 cup nonfat dry milk	Fri	☐☐☐☐
	6 oz. calcium-added orange juice	Sat	☐☐☐☐
	1 cup collard greens		
	1 1/2 cups cooked kale, mustard/turnip greens		
	1 3/4 cups broccoli		
	2 corn tortillas		
	10 dried figs		
	3 cups cooked dried beans (navy, pinto, Great northern)		
	Snacks: almonds, filberts, peanuts, dried fruit		

2+	**Vitamin C Foods**		
	1/2 grapefruit	Sun	☐☐☐☐
	1/2 cup grapefruit or orange juice (2 t concentrate)	Mon	☐☐☐☐
	2 small oranges	Tues	☐☐☐☐
	1/2 cup papaya, strawberries	Wed	☐☐☐☐
	1/4 small cantaloupe	Thurs	☐☐☐☐
	1 1/3 cup blackberries, raspberries	Fri	☐☐☐☐
	1 1/2 large tomatoes	Sat	☐☐☐☐
	1 cup tomato juice (3/4 cup V8)		
	3/4 cup cooked cauliflower		
	2/3 cup cooked broccoli		
	1/2 small red or green pepper		
	3 cups raw spinach		

3 or more (one raw) variety	**Green Leafy/Yellow Fruits & Vegetables** 1/8 cantaloupe 2 large fresh/dried apricots 1 large nectarine or yellow peach 1 t canned unsweetened pumpkin 1/3 cup cooked beet greens 3/4 cup cooked broccoli or turnip greens 1/2 raw carrot (1/3 cup if cooked) 8-10 leaves dark green leafy lettuce 1/2 cup raw spinach (1/4 cup if cooked) 1/4 cup cooked winter squash	Sun ☐☐☐☐ Mon ☐☐☐☐ Tues ☐☐☐☐ Wed ☐☐☐☐ Thurs ☐☐☐☐ Fri ☐☐☐☐ Sat ☐☐☐☐
2 or more	**Other Fruits and Vegetables** 1 apple or small banana 1/2 cup applesauce, unsweetened 6-7 asparagus spears 3/4 cup green beans 2/3 cup blueberries, zucchini 2/3 cup brussels sprouts 2/3 cup grapes 1 cup fresh mushrooms 1 medium white peach or pear 1 slice fresh pineapple, or unsweetened canned 1 medium potato	Sun ☐☐☐☐ Mon ☐☐☐☐ Tues ☐☐☐☐ Wed ☐☐☐☐ Thurs ☐☐☐☐ Fri ☐☐☐☐ Sat ☐☐☐☐
2 ½ full or 5 half or less max: 45 g or 405 calories	**High Fat Foods Half Servings** 1 oz cheese 1 1/2 oz. skim mozzarella 1 1/2 t light cream 1 t heavy whipping cream 2 t whipped cream 2 t sour cream 1 t cream cheese 1 cup 2%/whole milk (1 cup whole milk yogurt) 1/2 cup ice cream 1 t light margarine 1 t peanut butter 1/2 cup white sauce (1/3 cup Hollandaise sauce) 1 egg 2 cookies, muffins, cake 7 oz. light meat turkey/chicken, no skin 3 1/2 oz. dark meat turkey/chicken, no skin 3 oz. canned tuna	*Each box equals* *One-half serving* Sun ☐☐☐☐☐☐☐ Mon ☐☐☐☐☐☐☐ Tues ☐☐☐☐☐☐☐ Wed ☐☐☐☐☐☐☐ Thurs ☐☐☐☐☐☐☐ Fri ☐☐☐☐☐☐☐ Sat ☐☐☐☐☐☐☐
(Calculate this according to your desired weight and calorie intake)	**Full Servings** 1 t vegetable oil, margarine, mayonnaise, or butter 2 t regular salad dressing 3-6 oz. lean meat 3/4 cup tuna salad	Sun ☐☐ Mon ☐☐ Tues ☐☐ Wed ☐☐ Thurs ☐☐ Fri ☐☐ Sat ☐☐
some	**Iron-Rich Foods** beef, liver (infrequently), collards, kale, turnip greens, pumpkin, potatoes in skin, spinach, legumes, blackstrap molasses, dried fruits	

Section 5
Fitness

Exercise

WHY SHOULD YOU EXERCISE?

You know those warnings on the side of cigarettes: "The Surgeon General says this product is hazardous to your health" (or something close to that). Did you know that the surgeon general himself has listed in an official report that the lack of exercise is hazardous to your health? He has. In fact, exercise is one of the greatest well-being inducers you can find, often better than medicines, herbs, therapies, and surgeries.

So why don't we exercise then? If we know it's good for us and if we know we'll feel better about life in general, why don't we get up and get moving?

Usually basic inertia is the answer. An object that is not moving will not move without another

CATCH A CLUE

Remember the Library

So many of the new diet plans come in the form of best-selling books that can run you upwards of $25.00 a pop.

Remember to go to the library first. While you feel like you're making a commitment to better yourself by laying down that money, the truth is you don't better yourself until you use the information. And we all know how much of our hard-earned money is sitting on a bookshelf collecting dust.

Check it out. Check it out. Check it out.

force. It takes a lot of effort to change a sedentary (sitting around and *not* moving) lifestyle. It also takes time, and time is something that none of us has a surplus of. So in order for us to take out time for something that is not easy, we have to really believe in the payoff at the end. But here's the kicker: We don't really believe in the payoff until we take the effort to make the time. It's sort of a circle, isn't it?

And that is really why we should exercise. We need to get up and get going and see the difference we can make so that we can have the reason and the momentum to live a fit and fabulous life. We should care enough about ourselves to want to live long and to want to enjoy the life that we live.

Why should you exercise?
- Because your body will function more efficiently.
- Because you'll feel better.
- Because you'll keep your weight under better control.
- Because you'll probably live longer.
- Because you'll probably keep the whole rest of your life in better order.
- Because, chances are, you'll smile more.

There are more reasons, but, for this list, that's why you should exercise.

WHAT ARE THE BENEFITS?

We know that exercise affects our lives in positive ways. Exercise is probably the most ignored health serum there is. When we exercise consistently, we decrease our risk of heart disease and increase our potential for long lives. When we exercise consistently, we enable our bodies to function more efficiently and our bones to grow in strength and carry us longer and better.

Exercise functions not only as a health and well-being inducer but also as a mood pick-me-up. Besides that, it improves our perspective about life. When we go to the trouble to exercise our bodies, we are more likely to do the other things that will keep us healthy, like eating well.

Here's a list. Pick whichever benefits matter the most to you and will get you moving.
- Exercise strengthens bones.
- Exercise protects against disease.
- Exercise relieves premenstrual discomfort.

WIDE ANGLE

Yo-Yo Dieting

The general consensus about the damages of yo-yo dieting seems to have changed over the years. Not too long ago most people felt that the more their weight went up and down the harder it was to lose weight and the harder it was to control their metabolism. More often than not these days, dieticians and nutritionists are saying that going back and forth with your weight (for instance, that same twenty pounds lost twenty times) doesn't harm your physical ability to lose weight. It may hinder your drive and ambition though. "Can I do it one more time? Will I just gain it back?"

So what does that mean for you? It means keep trying even if you've gained it back. It means go ahead and try whether you feel like you're ready to go the whole ten miles or not. There are so many "reasons" that hold us back from dieting. Don't let the fear of yo-yo dieting be one of them.

- Exercise eases menopause.
- Exercise raises your metabolism (and so the rate at which you burn calories).
- Exercise often raises your sense of well-being and self-esteem.
- Exercise increases your chances of losing weight.
- Exercise increases your chances of keeping lost weight off.
- Exercise helps you eat less.
- Exercise protects against muscle loss.
- Exercise decreases many symptoms of aging.
- Exercise aids circulation (including circulation to the brain, which increases mental alertness).
- Exercise pumps more oxygen into your body tissues.
- Exercise helps your body respond to insulin.
- Exercise gives you a sense of control over your own well-being.

GET STARTED

Here are a few old favorite exercises to get you started:

Resting position: Stand straight with your feet shoulder-width apart and your arms out at your sides at shoulder height.

1. Stand up straight in resting position. Taking in a big breath, stretch your arms up toward the ceiling, lifting your whole body up, from your toes to your head. Then release your breath and lower your arms back to shoulder height. (Four repetitions.)
2. Stand up straight in resting position. Twist your upper body at the waist so that you are turning from right to left. You should feel the pull in your waist and sides. (Eight repetitions.)
3. Stand up straight in resting position. Bend over at the waist and touch your left foot (or as close to it as possible) with your right hand. Stand up straight again. Repeat, but this time touch your right foot with your left hand. You should feel the pull in your waist, back, and thighs. (Eight repetitions per side.)
4. Stand beside a chair or doorpost in resting position. Hold on for balance. Bend one leg at the knee and then lift the leg out to the side. You should feel the pull in the back of your thighs and buttocks. (Eight repetitions per leg.)
5. Lay down on your back and bend your knees. Put your hands at each side of your head. Raise your upper body toward the ceiling just enough to get your shoulder blades off the floor. Then lower your upper body back down to the floor. (Eight repetitions.)

6. Still on your back, raise your legs up to sitting position. Bicycle your legs by first lowering your right leg almost to the floor, then raising it again as you lower your left leg almost to the floor. (Eight repetitions per leg.)

7. Before you stand back up, roll over onto all fours. Lift your left leg so that your foot is pointing toward the ceiling. Lower it back down so that your knee is on the floor. Lift your right leg so that your right foot is pointing toward the ceiling. Lower it back down so that your right knee is on the floor. (Eight repetitions per leg.)

8. Finish up by standing again in resting position and doing four more deep-breathing arm lifts.

It's just a start and nothing brand spanking new. Take fifteen minutes and start moving your body and stretching those muscles.

Exercise + Dieting = Much Better Success

As far as dieting goes, you are setting yourself up for success when you combine exercise with a low-fat, high-fiber, moderate protein and carb food plan. Think of it this way: You are setting out to climb a mountain so you gather all the appropriate tools into your backpack, throw the backpack on your back, and head up the mountain using nothing more than a pair of leather gloves for grip.

That's crazy! You've picked the right task. You've set about the right direction. You know what you want to accomplish. But instead of using the tools that are at your disposal to help you accomplish your goals, they are just weighing you down. That's what it's like to diet without exercising.

It's great to eat low calories or low fat foods, but it's better if you enlist your body's support. You can do that by raising your body's metabolism through exercise. You probably already know this, but your metabolism is the speed at which your body processes everything. The higher your metabolism, the more calories you burn in a smaller amount of time. So a high metabolism is a good thing. Exercising regularly raises your metabolism. No one will disagree with that. This means every change you make in your food plan, everything you deprive yourself of, every sacrifice you make will be worth more because your body is using up what you are giving it even more quickly than before you exercised.

What Is a Perfect Ten?

In our culture a perfect ten is almost an impossible goal. Our perfect tens are splattered across magazine covers. They are the best of the best. They are sometimes natural beauties, the fortunate, the good-gene-induced. They are often the plastic-surgery-molded and the collagen-pumped-up. Because we see them on magazine covers, we assume that they are the norm. But actually the people that our culture calls perfect tens are usually the exception to the rule. (Some even say as few as one person in forty-thousand has "model looks.") So if they are the exception, what is the rule?

Most of the people you know are the rule. *You* are the rule.

There's a big difference between (1) trying to measure up to unrealistic expectations, and (2) trying to be the best you can be. You might

THE BIBLE SAYS

Scripture That Helps

Whenever you hear someone talk about exercise you often hear them use the following Scriptures. Sometimes our only response to these passages is guilt and shame. Give up the guilt and shame, but remember these nuggets from the Word of God as you're sweating to the oldies (or whatever else you might sweat to. . .).

We honor God when we care for ourselves.

"Do you not know that your body is a temple of the Holy Spirit, who is in you, whom you have received from God? You are not your own; you were bought at a price. Therefore honor God with your body" (1 Corinthians 6:19–20).

(This advice was written in the context of sexual sin but gives us a principle that applies to a lot of areas of our lives.)

"Therefore, I urge you, brothers, in view of God's mercy, to offer your bodies as living sacrifices, holy and pleasing to God—this is your spiritual act of worship. Do not conform any longer to the pattern of this world, but be transformed by the renewing of your mind. Then you will be able to test and approve what God's will is—his good, pleasing and perfect will" (Romans 12:1–2).

diet and exercise. You might lose weight. And guess what? You probably still won't look like those women with the smooth, taut legs (airbrushed) or the guys with the defined ribs (drawn in with charcoal).

It's a difficult reality to face: No matter how hard you work, you still have your own body. You can make it better. You can tone those muscles. You can even get some plastic surgery. But it's still your body. If you're short, you'll still be short. If your family tends toward heavy upper arms, you might not ever get rid of that entirely. Your basic body shape will very well still be your basic body shape.

So what do you do with that? What should your expectations be? What yardstick has the measurements that you should strive for?

Your expectations in losing weight should really be the same as your expectations in life:

- to be fit
- to make the most of your best attributes
- to make peace with the parts of yourself that don't match up with the magazine covers

BODY SHAPES

So besides eating it, what does fruit have to do with dieting? When you're talking about body shapes, fruits can mean a lot. The most popular fruit-labeled body shapes are the apple and the pear.

A person with an apple body shape is a person who gains weight in the upper portion of his body instead of or as well as in the lower half. Men are most prone to this body shape because they don't gain in the hips and legs as much as women. For them it is the "beer guts" and the big bellies.

The particular danger of this kind of weight gain is the fat around the heart. People (men and women) whose bodies are apple shaped have a greater risk of heart disease. Women whose bodies are apple shaped also have a greater risk of endometrial cancer and breast cancer.

When people (men or women) tend to store their fat below the waist in their hips and thighs, their bodies are described as pear shaped. The good thing about being pear shaped is that the fat is not gathering around your heart. You can figure out the bad things about being pear shaped.

But whatever your body shape or your metabolism or your exercise regimen, the important thing is that you can always improve what needs improving.

Cardiovascular Fitness

Hey, all you couch potatoes! We hate to break the news to you, but cardiovascular fitness is not achieved sitting down. You've got to get up and get moving. Not sure what cardiovascular fitness is or even if you want to be fit? Well, don't change that dial. We're here to inform and interest you. Fitness is fun!

WHAT IS CARDIOVASCULAR EXERCISE?

It sounds so technical, so scientific, but cardiovascular exercise is any exercise that uses large muscle groups (like your legs and arms), increases your heart rate to sixty to ninety percent of your maximum heart rate and can be maintained for at least twenty minutes. Not sure how to figure your maximum heart rate? Read on.

FIGURING YOUR MAXIMUM HEART RATE

Maximum Heart Rate Per Minute = 220 minus your age
Example:

220–30 years = 190 beats per minute

For safety's sake, you should not exercise at an intensity that will raise your heart rate above your maximum heart rate.

Cardiovascular a.k.a. Aerobic Exercises

If your idea of exercising is running across the street or chasing your toddler, think again. Aerobic literally means *with oxygen*. Aerobic exercise is when you exercise at a level where you are not deprived of oxygen, like in sprinting. So for all of you who thought you could get fit by sprinting for a minute every other day—you might get faster, but you won't get aerobically fit. Nor does aerobic fitness come with biking for thirty minutes so slowly that you almost fall off your bike. You have to exercise at the proper intensity for the right amount of time for it to be considered aerobic exercise and of any benefit. Here's a list of exercises that if done at the proper intensity are considered aerobic:
• Running
• Swimming

- Walking
- Bicycling
- Cross-country skiing
- Hiking
- Aerobic dancing
- Speed skating
- Rowing
- Rollerblading

Other activities that count as aerobic if played well and without much stopping include:
- Soccer
- Basketball
- Racquetball
- Paddleball

GAINING CARDIOVASCULAR FITNESS

It only makes sense that you gain cardiovascular fitness by doing cardiovascular exercise. (We truly are rocket scientists!) But there really is more to it than that. It can get a little tricky, so stay alert. There are four factors that must be considered if fitness is to be obtained. They are frequency of exercise, intensity of exercise, duration of exercise, and type of activity. Fortunately the American College of Sports Medicine has made some recommendations for developing and maintaining cardiovascular fitness utilizing these factors. The four factors are:

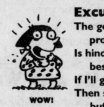

Excuses
The good exercising produces,
Is hindered by my best excuses.
If I'll get off my duff,
Then soon I'll be buff,
And fit for all kinds of new uses.

wow!

Frequency of exercise: You should exercise three to five days a week. Nonconsecutive days are recommended to allow recovery from the exercise sessions.

Intensity of exercise: The exercise should be hard enough that your heart rate is between sixty and ninety percent of your maximum heart rate. Since intensity is measured by heart rate, an increase in heart rate equals an increase in intensity. Note that on the average, maximum heart rates decrease by about ten beats per minute per decade of life. So as you age, your intensity should decrease.

Duration of exercise: The exercise should be performed continuously at the proper intensity for twenty to sixty minutes per session. Duration is dependent on the intensity of the activity. So if you are exercising at a lower intensity, you need to exercise for a longer period of time. For example: If you are walking at sixty percent of your max heart rate, you would need to walk for a longer period to achieve the same fitness level of running at eighty percent of your max heart rate.

Type of Activity: Any of the exercises listed on the previous pages under cardiovascular exercises would qualify.

Body Image/ Body Reality

THE BOTTOM LINE Our body image is about more than what we see when we look in the mirror. It's about how we feel about what we see. Do you see thighs that are way bigger than you want them to be? Your body image is what you decide about yourself because of those thighs. Do you decide that you are totally unattractive? Do you decide that you will never find a mate? Or do you decide that your thighs are just bigger than you want them to be?

Don't allow the mirror to make decisions for you about your potential in life or your worth as a person. We are all more than the sum total of our parts.

Remember that your body is more than something to look at. It functions for you. It keeps you alive. It carries you places and allows you to relate to other people. Your body serves you well in many ways.

WARMING UP AND WARMING DOWN

If you're thinking about hopping out of bed tomorrow, throwing on your running duds, and expecting to dart out your door at eighty-five percent of your maximum heart rate, think again. Not only is it unwise, but you could hurt yourself. Let us tell you a little secret that will keep injuries at bay and help your sleeping muscles wake up. It's called a warm-up.

Prior to any aerobic activity, take several minutes to exercise slowly to get the blood flowing to your muscles. Many people choose to warm up doing the same aerobic activity, only at a much slower pace. For instance, bike slowly before getting into your regular biking pace. Walk before jogging. Do some calisthenics before swimming. Whatever you do, make sure it's using the same large muscles you'll be using in your aerobic activity. Just as important as the warm-up is the cool-down which follows the exercise. The cool-down should include slowing your exercise pace for several minutes followed by stretching exercises. The cool-down helps prevent blood from pooling in your extremities, which reduces the chance of dizziness and fainting, and also reduces muscle soreness from the workout. So the next time you decide to end your running workout, remember to take an extra minute or two to walk or jog slowly and then stretch your legs. It could mean the difference between your foot or your face hitting the pavement.

BENEFITS OF CARDIOVASCULAR FITNESS

The benefits of cardiovascular fitness are outstanding. In fact, exercising is so beneficial, it's surprising someone would even consider *not* exercising. Here's a list of benefits from exercising:

1. Decreases risk of suffering heart attack and stroke. Exercise helps decrease blood pressure and lowers cholesterol—two major contributing factors affecting one's chance for heart attack or stroke.
2. Controls weight. Exercising burns calories. The more calories you're expending (and hopefully not taking them back in), the more weight you will lose.
3. Strengthens the heart and lowers resting heart rate. Your heart is a muscle and just as weight lifting helps strengthen your muscles, aerobic exercise helps strengthen your heart. A slow resting heart rate in a healthy person is the sign of a strong, efficient heart. It can push more blood with each beat than the heart of someone with a higher resting heart rate.
4. Increases lung volume. Just as a trained individual's heart becomes stronger, aerobic exercise enables your lungs to expand to a greater capacity.
5. Builds and strengthens bone. Weight-bearing exercises, such as running or walking, help build and strengthen bones, which aids in the prevention of osteoporosis.
6. Increases endurance capacity. Soon you'll be able to exercise for longer periods and going up that flight of stairs won't wind you like it used to, because your endurance capacity has increased.
7. Slows down the aging process. Believe it or not, it really does! As we age, we lose muscle mass, gain more fat, our bones weaken, and we lose flexibility. Aerobic exercise counteracts each of those problems directly.

Now if those aren't enough reasons to get out there and start exercising, you must need a swift kick to get moving. Even though you won't receive a certificate of accomplishment when you do become fit, you will notice some other distinct benefits:

- improved sleep
- increased self-discipline
- improved self-esteem
- character development
- stress relief

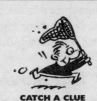

CATCH A CLUE

Finding Your Pulse:

There is a short-cut to taking your pulse for a minute. Instead, count your pulse for six seconds. Multiply that number by ten and you have your heart rate for a minute.

For example: If you counted eight heart beats in six seconds, you'd have a pulse rate of eighty beats per minute.

While there are a ton of benefits to aerobic exercise, they are not the only reasons we should exercise our body. God has given us our bodies as a gift, and they are also the dwelling places for His Spirit. We must take care of what God has given us, and we can do that by staying fit.

Choosing an Aerobic Program

So you've decided that it's time to start exercising, but you're not interested in running a marathon or doing the Ironman Triathlon; you just want to get into shape. Instead of jumping into any old exercise just to be doing something, consider the following questions. Your answers will mold your exercise program into one you like and should have success with.

Questions to ask yourself:

How much time can I commit? Take a good look at your day and any responsibilities and involvements you have. If after work you become the human taxi to and from your children's many activities, then rush home to make dinner, followed by time spent helping with homework and giving baths, then it is logical to commit time in the morning before work. Maybe you can carve out a thirty-minute walk on your lunch hour. Or try going for a jog after the kids get on the bus for school. Whatever your situation, decide how much time you can commit to working out. Don't forget to allow for time to get ready before and after your workout.

What are my likes and dislikes? Do you despise running but just love to swim? Would you rather not get sweaty? Do you like the feeling of speed and wind blowing through your hair? Do you hate getting up early in the morning? Would you rather work out inside than outside? Identifying your likes and dislikes will help tailor your exercise program to your specific needs.

What goal do I want to accomplish? Ask yourself whether you are looking to lose weight, gain overall fitness, or train for an event like a five-kilometer run. Determining a goal gives definition to your program.

Exercise Won't:

1. Win you a million dollars.
2. Make your straight hair curly.
3. Heal your hangnail.
4. Whiten your teeth.
5. Make your boss give you a raise.

WOW!

How much discipline do I have? Let's be realistic here. If you tend to quit activities after a week, then be sure to tailor your program and goals so you can stick with them. An exercise program does no good if you don't follow through with it.

What are my health risks? Determine if there are any issues or risks that need to be considered when creating your program. For instance, do you have a family history of heart problems? See a doctor first. Do you have any injuries or past problems like a bad back or knee? Stick with low-impact exercise like swimming, biking, or walking. Do you suffer from asthma or allergies? Consider working out indoors.

Your answers to these questions determine what kind of program is appropriate for you.

But there are two important tips to keep in mind before starting your program:
1. *See a doctor before starting any kind of exercise program,* especially if you have a risk of heart disease or history of injuries.

2. *Don't buy any exercise equipment at the beginning of your program.* Try renting or borrowing that bike, stair-stepper, or rowing machine before plunking down the cash to own it. Don't spend a lot of money just to find out you would rather jog outside than run on a treadmill, or you'll be stuck with an expensive clothes-drying rack.

CROSS-TRAINING

No matter how much you like an activity, most people get tired of doing the same workout day in and day out. But there is hope. You can wipe off that glazed look you get from running too much by *cross-*

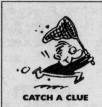

CATCH A CLUE

Cardiovascular Exercise Is Not:

1. Reaching for the TV remote control.
2. Shopping for fitness wear.
3. Watching aerobics on TV.
4. Going to a football game.
5. Brushing your teeth.

training, a fancy word for alternating activities. Go out and bike for one workout. Then try rollerblading or alternate with running. The idea is that you'll use different sets of muscles, have less overuse injuries, and you won't be as bored. So feel free to mix up the activities. Whatever you do, try and have fun. Getting into shape should not be a drag.

WORKOUT IDEAS

Maybe you like to exercise but have gotten stuck in a rut and need some creative ideas to spice up your workout life. Take another look at your day and see where you could make a change.

- Try walking on your lunch hour. Have access to a shower at work? Go for a jog over lunch. (Be sure to have a light snack about an hour before and eat lunch afterwards.)
- Bike to and from work. Or drive halfway to work, park your car, and bike the rest of the way. Reverse it for the commute home.
- Go for an early morning swim. It's truly an eye-opener!
- Try trail running.
- Join a gym, fitness center, or health club.
- Join a running or biking club.
- Sign up for a basketball league.
- Start an aerobics class.
- Take up speed skating.
- Buy a new exercise tape.
- Invest in a new exercise machine (after trying it out, of course).

STICKING WITH THE PROGRAM

Even though you've created your ideal exercise program, at first it *will* be hard to motivate yourself. You might literally have to drag yourself out to get started, but stick with the program. And trust us; it will get easier with time. Pretty soon you'll start to see benefits, like feeling better and sleeping better, that make all the discomfort and sweat worthwhile. Here are some tips to help you stick with your exercise program:

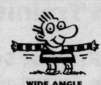

WIDE ANGLE

It Can Work Wonders

"Before I started exercising, I tended to sleep a lot and was often late wherever I went. My husband even had to call me after he got to work in the morning to make sure I had gotten out of bed and fed the kids breakfast! But after I had been exercising for several months, I became more disciplined and no longer needed the wake-up call. And now, I actually try to be early wherever I go."
—Laurel, Wayzata, Minnesota

1. Exercise with a buddy. Knowing that someone is expecting you to show up makes it harder to skip a workout. The "Oops, I just didn't have time to run today," excuse just doesn't cut it when your buddy is waiting for you down at the corner.
2. Make your program a habit. Habits are formed when you do something in threes. Start by exercising three days a week, then do it for three weeks, six weeks, three months, and so on.
3. Incorporate this program into your lifestyle. Don't just add it on to your daily routine; infuse it. Just like eating three meals a day, watching your favorite TV show every week, or following the same pattern to get ready in the morning, your program should become a part of your life.

THE BIBLE SAYS

Walking Temples

"Don't you know that your body is the temple of the Holy Spirit, who lives in you and was given to you by God? You do not belong to yourself, for God bought you with a high price. So you must honor God with your body" (1 Corinthians 6:19–20 NLT).

4. Work toward goals. Goals instigate initiative. No matter how small the goal, whether it's to be able to jog around the park or walk a mile, reaching a goal lifts one's self-esteem and breeds the desire for more success.

Strength Training

DIFFERENCE BETWEEN STRENGTH TRAINING AND AEROBIC EXERCISE

"Aren't I building my muscles by doing aerobic exercise?" It's a common question, and the answer unfortunately is *not exactly*. But there is an upside. Your muscles are gaining more strength than if you were just sitting at a desk or standing around, simply because you are using your muscles during your workout. But if you want to gain muscle strength, you need to lift weights or do resistance training.

BODY TYPES

Rather than tiptoe through the tulips as we enter the delicate territory of body typing, let's face it. Everyone is built a little different. Some of us have the classic bell or pear shape while others are built like a fence post or already look like they've been lifting

It's Hard Work

But exercise actually might help you find a date or even a mate! Read

WOW!

this true story and all you singles out there might start exercising today!

"I joined a running club because I wanted to have a group that would hold me accountable for exercising. I became good friends with a guy there, and we would often run next to each other so we could talk. Eventually he asked me out, and the rest is history—we got married, and now we're training for the Boston Marathon."
—Jane, St. Charles, Illinois

weights. Although you can't change your body type, you can work with it. Understanding the different body types and identifying your own will make your expectations of your strength training workout more realistic.

Body Types:

Mesomorph—These folks are characterized by a square body with prominent muscles. They are the "athletic"-looking body type.

Endomorph—These are the folks who are characterized by roundness and softness, and they have no muscle definition. Their body shape is often called a bell or pear with their abdomen being wider than their shoulders.

Ectomorph—These folks are characterized by leanness. Their bones are small and their muscles thin, thus the name *thin as a rail*.

No one falls solely into one category, but instead exhibits characteristics from all three categories. Understanding which characteristics you exhibit will guide your goals and temper your workout expectations. For instance, if you show more characteristics of the ectomorph category, then you will have trouble acquiring big, bulky muscles, because it is just not your body type. Or if you show more characteristics of the endomorph category, it will take

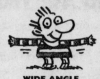

You Never Know

"After a year and a half of wasting time sitting through my kids' speed-skating practices, I decided I could put that time to good use and get in shape. So I borrowed some skates and started speed skating too. Not only have I gotten in shape, but I've started competing at the master's level and actually won some races!"
—**Nancy, Milwaukee, Wisconsin**

longer and much effort to show signs of muscular definition. Knowing this about yourself will keep you from getting frustrated if it takes longer than expected to see signs of being in shape. Those in the mesomorph category tend to look athletic, but are not necessarily in shape. But keep in mind, how you look is not an indication of physical fitness. Whether or not you tend to look athletic doesn't mean you are.

TONING VS. BODY BUILDING

If you're looking to build some muscle strength without the rippling abdominals and eye-popping biceps, then strength training is for you. But if you're interested in losing the flab that hangs on the backs of your arms and jiggles when you lift them over your head, then muscle toning is what you should look into. Either way, you need some equipment.

HOME VS. GYM EQUIPMENT

For all you strength trainers, it's best to start at a gym or health club because you get an idea of what weights you really need before spending a lot of money on your own. Plus the trainers provide pointers on the correct lifting form. You want to be sure you're doing the exercises correctly to avoid injury. After getting comfortable with the weights you use, then consider buying. If you are planning to tone your muscles, you can also join a gym, but there are some great resistive exercises done with tubing that you can do at home.

QUESTIONS TO ASK YOURSELF

Need some help deciding what is best for you? Consider the following questions:

- *What do I want to gain? Muscle bulk, muscle strength, or muscle tone?*
- *Do I have time for both weight training/resistance training and aerobic exercise?*
- *How much money do I want to spend? Am I willing to join a health club or use some tubing and simple weights at home?*

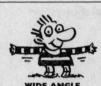

WIDE ANGLE

Keep It Fresh

"I tend to get bored easily if I do the same exercise a lot, so I alternate different activities. If it's too hot out, I'll go swimming. The next day I might bike. I'll even take the dog for a long walk or jog with the baby in the stroller. Mixing it up keeps me interested in working out."
—Kirsten, Toledo, Ohio

READY TO LIFT

You've bought the right attire, you've set aside the time to lift, and you're ready to go. Since free weights are the best route to building bigger muscles, you need dumbbells and the weights that have a bar and interchangeable weights at either end. Then there's the lingo. Weight lifters talk in terms of sets and reps (a.k.a. repetitions). That's how many times you should lift the weight. If you want to build muscle endurance then follow the lifting sequence of two to three sets of fifteen repetitions. That means you lift the weight fifteen times, take a short thirty-second break, lift it again fifteen more times, followed by another break and then fifteen more repetitions. The weight should be heavy enough that it's challenging, but light enough that you can lift it fifteen times without stopping. This sequence should be completed for every muscle or muscle group.

If you want to build muscle strength, the lifting sequence is three sets of ten repetitions. But the weight should be heavy enough that the last two to three repetitions of every set are almost too heavy to lift. Strength training works on the overload principle. This states that a muscle will gain strength only when it performs for a given time at its maximal strength capacity. So you need to lift as heavy as possible to gain strength.

MAJOR MUSCLE GROUPS

The top five major muscle groups to work are:

1. legs—quadriceps, hamstrings, and calf muscles
2. arms—biceps and triceps
3. chest—pectoral muscles
4. back—latissimus dorsi and rhomboids
5. abdominals

HITTING THE GYM

Ever walked into a health club and wondered why there are so many different weight machines and ways to lift weights? How do you possibly choose which ones to use? It all depends on your goal. If you're looking to gain muscle bulk, then free weights are your best bet. If you're looking to gain muscle strength, endurance, and a smaller amount of bulk, choose the machines called Nautilus, Eagle, Cybex, etc. These provide consistent resistance throughout your muscle's full range of motion during the lift, whereas free weights only strengthen the weakest point in your lifting range of motion.

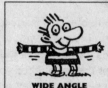

WIDE ANGLE

Accountability Helps

"Frequently my alarm would go off and all I would want to do was roll over and go back to sleep. But knowing Karin would be waiting for me to go walking always got me going. I knew I couldn't let her down."
—Laura, Franklin, Tennessee

TRAINING TIPS

Keep in mind:
- Your muscles need a recovery day in between lifting days. Because you're actually breaking down muscle while lifting, you need a day to allow your muscles to rebuild and recover. They are actually building their strength on the recovery days, so be sure to take those days.
- Be sure to have someone with you who is trained to show you how to lift properly. Risk of injury is very high, so make sure you're doing things right.
- Lift with a partner. Some of the exercises require a spotter—like the bench press. Plus it's just plain smart to have someone there in case you are lifting a heavy weight and need help finishing a set. You'd hate to be trapped in your basement with a two-hundred-pound bar on your chest and no way to lift it off!

- Remember to lift after warming up. If you're doing some form of aerobic exercise, lift afterwards. If not, be sure to do some calisthenics before lifting to get the blood flowing to your muscles and avoid injury.

MUSCLE TONING

So you're feeling a little flabby and ready to do something about it, but weight lifting conjures up images of you standing in a line of people flexing your bulging muscles for a panel of judges. Not looking to get that extreme? Then we've got the routine for you. Fortunately, it's relatively inexpensive too! All you need is yourself and some resistance tubing (a four- to five-foot-long strand of rubber tubing) or resistance bands (an inch-wide circular band about eight inches long) which can be purchased at your local athletic store, and you're set to tone your muscles. Although you won't be gaining bulk from these exercises, you can still work on strength and endurance. The lifting sequence is the same as in weight lifting. For strength, do three sets of ten repetitions. For endurance, do two to three sets of fifteen repetitions. For exercise techniques, read on.

SIMPLE EFFECTIVE TECHNIQUES

Since we're sure you don't want to leave any muscle untoned, we've got some exercises to work the five major muscle groups. Be sure to alternate arms or legs between sets.

Bicep curl: Stand with one end of tubing anchored under your foot and grasp the other end with your hand. With palm facing away from body, lift hand up to shoulder as you bend your elbow and then slowly extend arm back to side. Make sure tubing is tight enough that you have resistance throughout the whole movement.

Tricep curl: Stand with one end of tubing anchored under your foot and grasp the other end with your hand. Keeping arm straight, lift arm backwards away from hip and then slowly return arm to side.

Rowing: Knot the tubing in the middle. Place the knot at chest level in the door frame and close the door. Now grasp the other end with both hands and step away from door so tubing is taut and your arms are extended at chest level. With both arms, pull tubing backwards until elbows are bent behind your back, and then slowly reextend arms. Be sure to keep arms parallel with the floor at all times. This exercise works your back muscles.

The following exercises require a resistance or tension band.

Knee extensions: Sit in a chair with the band around both your ankles. Holding one leg in place, lift and straighten the other leg against the resistance of the band and then slowly bend leg back to original position.

Leg curls: Lie on stomach with knees bent and the band around your ankles. Keeping one leg bent, straighten the other leg down toward the floor and then bend it slowly back to the original position.

The following exercises don't require any tubing or band.

Squats: Stand with feet shoulder-width apart and toes slightly pointing out. With hands on your hips, bend knees to about a forty-five-degree angle and then straighten back up.

Calf raises: Stand with toes on a step and heels hanging off the edge. Lift yourself up until you're standing on tiptoes, then slowly lower until heels are below the step. Keep toes in contact with step at all times. Continue to alternate the raising and lowering. To make this more difficult, try it on one leg at a time.

Sit-ups: Lie on back with knees bent and hands behind your head. While looking up at the ceiling, slowly lift head, neck, and shoulders off the ground and then slowly lower back down to the ground.

Push-ups: In the prone position, support your body weight with your hands (placed on the ground shoulder-width apart) and with your toes or knees (yes, girl push-ups are just as effective!), slowly bend elbows until your nose touches the ground and then slowly push yourself up by straightening your arms.

The great thing about these exercises is that they are inexpensive, you can do them anywhere (tubing travels great), and you really don't break a sweat unless it's over ninety degrees outside! So what are you waiting for? Let's get toning!

wow!

Looks Aren't Everything

"When I competed in my first triathlon, I thought I was in pretty good shape, until I got passed on the run by someone who looked like he had never worked out! He hardly had any muscle definition at all and seemed a little overweight, but he sure could run fast, and he beat me!"
—**Nate, Chicago, Illinois**

A Word about Spot Reducing

Who doesn't have an area on their body that seems like it needs some extra help? It's where the fat tends to settle (forever, it seems)—the inner thighs, the outer thighs, your derriere, or the backs of your arms. But how do you get rid of it? It's the ten-million-dollar question. We hate to burst your bubble, but it's not spot reducing. You might have heard of spot reducing. You might have even tried it. The idea behind it is for you to pinpoint a trouble spot and do exercises specifically for that area that supposedly melt away the fat. It seems logical, and it makes you feel like you're actually doing something to help that area, but we're here to share the truth. Spot reducing *will* tone the muscle underneath the fat, but it *won't* get rid of the fat. Only a combination of aerobic exercise, restricting calories, and toning exercises will help you lose fat and slim down those trouble spots.

Muscle Gain vs. Weight Loss

If after a few weeks of doing aerobic exercise and lifting weights or doing resistive exercises, you jump on the scale and find you actually weigh more than when you started exercising, don't get frustrated and throw this book and your program out the window. There is a logical reason. Lifting weights and doing resistive exercises builds muscle—and here's

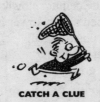

CATCH A CLUE

Gym Etiquette Faux Pas

1. Wearing dark socks with white shoes
2. Asking someone to help you lift the weight
3. Constantly staring at yourself in the mirrors
4. Dropping a dumbbell on someone's toe
5. Striking up a conversation with someone while they're lifting a weight

the kicker—*muscle actually weighs more than fat*. You will probably see an *increase* in weight as your body is transitioning from less fat to more muscle, but that is a good thing. Toned muscle burns more calories than untoned muscles or fat, so the more muscle you have, the more calories you're burning. So don't throw in the towel when you see a larger number on the scale than you'd expected. Stick with the program, and you'll soon get the results you want.

STRETCHING

While it's tempting to lift weights or do resistive exercises and then hit the showers, it is not a good idea. Lifting weights actually shortens the muscles, so do some stretching exercises afterwards to increase flexibility and decrease your chances of injury. Here are some tips for proper stretching techniques:

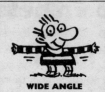

Strength vs. Endurance Training

Strength Training Sequence: Three sets of ten repetitions, three days a week
Endurance Training Sequence: Two to three sets of fifteen repetitions, three days a week

1. Do a static stretch. Rather than bobbing or bouncing in the stretching position, hold the stretch position without moving. Bouncing can cause tiny tears in the muscles.
2. Hold the stretch for *at least* thirty seconds. The muscle needs time for its fibers to stretch. Anything less than thirty seconds is not enough time for that to happen.
3. Stretch each muscle group two to three times. Hold the stretch for thirty seconds, take a fifteen-second break and then stretch again for thirty seconds. Follow up with another break and thirty-second stretch.

MAINTAINING MUSCLE FITNESS

If you don't mind lifting weights or just love your resistance program, that's great. But we're sure there are some of you who are wondering if you're going to be lifting weights three days a week for the rest of your life in order to maintain strength. The answer is no. The most difficult phase of your strength training program is the *development* of strength. Once this has been accomplished, it is relatively easy to maintain. Hitting the weights once a week, provided you're lifting the heaviest weights possible for you, will help you maintain about seventy percent of your strength. To maintain full strength, you need to keep up with the three days a week routine. But hey! Some strength is sometimes better than no strength!

REMEMBER: It's easy to become obsessed with how we look and the kind of shape we're in. When we do, we make an idol—a god—out of ourselves or exercise, and God is replaced. We need to be careful that our outward appearance does not become more important than the condition of our hearts. For in the end, we will be judged by our hearts, not how we look.

Lifetime Fitness

LONG-TERM HEALTH

As depressing as it sounds, lack of exercise and low levels of physical fitness are very important risk factors for disease and early death. That's not to say that you have to be extremely athletic or do large volumes of exercise. If you don't feel like training for a marathon, it's OK. Moderate levels of exercise and fitness offer major health benefits like a decrease in heart disease, diabetes, high blood pressure, some cancers, osteoporosis, and, of course, obesity. But the key is to do moderate levels of exercise throughout your whole life.

KEYS TO LONG-TERM HEALTH

- Mix aerobic exercise with simple muscle-strengthening exercises. Important muscle tissue and muscle strength is lost as we age. But research shows it's never too late to rebuild and strengthen muscle with exercise.
- Establish good eating patterns and stick with them. Good nutrition is habit-forming and your quality of diet becomes more important the older you get.
- Limit fat, cholesterol, and sodium in your diet to help prevent cardiovascular disease.
- Maintain a balance between energy consumed and energy expended. Balance physical activity and a healthy diet.

TOTAL FITNESS PLAN

When creating your long-term fitness plan, don't strictly limit yourself to the physical aspect. It is important to live a balanced life by developing the mental, emotional, and spiritual aspects of your life as well. It's important to keep our bodies in shape to live healthfully as we age, but we need to be spending daily time in God's Word and in prayer to keep us spiritually healthy.

TREAT YOUR BODY LIKE A FINE MACHINE

1. Schedule regular maintenance checkups. These include physicals, dental checks, screening for disorders that you're at a high risk for,

and vision and hearing screenings.
2. Keep the engine clean. Avoid high-fat diets and smoking. Use your cardiovascular system often.
3. Give the engine an adequate and appropriate energy source. Maintain a balanced diet, and supplement with vitamins when necessary.
4. Work the engine; don't let it freeze up. Exercise both the mind and muscles.
5. Keep safety a priority when operating. Get flu shots, wear seat belts and glasses, avoid alcohol, and practice defensive driving.

KUDOS FOR EXERCISE

Exercise is associated with:
- More effective stress management
- Fewer sleep disorders
- Enlightened mental outlook
- Reduced loneliness
- Lowered depression and anxiety

SETTING GOALS AND PRIORITIES

Setting goals and priorities for lifetime fitness is crucial if you're really going to maintain it over the long haul. As you proceed through life, you will need to look at your schedule and rework your goals. How you stay fit will probably change throughout the years, but don't get discouraged if at certain times in your life you're not in the shape you were in when you were twenty. Stay motivated, and you'll reap the benefits of healthy living in the end.

STAYING MOTIVATED

Staying motivated to maintain fitness over the long haul is a difficult thing to do. The dropout rates are higher for people who:
1. Take up a vigorous activity rather than a moderate activity.
2. Do "too much too soon" and get injured or sore.
3. Have family and friends who don't exercise.
4. Don't believe they can stick with a regular exercise program.
5. Have so many family/social/job-related activities going on that they can't find time to exercise.
6. Believe it's "too late" to get in better shape.

We've come up with some solutions to three different barriers to getting started on your long-term fitness plan. Read on.

Problem #1: No time
Solution: Sneak exercise into your day.

- Get up thirty minutes earlier and exercise before breakfast.
- Walk or bike to and from work.
- Take the stairs instead of the elevator.
- Make the most out of an activity you do already (i.e., walking). Simply increase the frequency and pace.
- In the evening, jump on your exercycle, or use a stair-climber or treadmill while you watch the news or a favorite TV show.
- Take a family walk in the evening.

Body Sculpting

"My trouble spot has always been my inner thighs. When I heard about spot reducing, I became so motivated to slim them down that I did the leg exercises twice a day. I was pretty surprised when one day I put on my jeans and they felt tight in the legs. Lo and behold, my leg muscles had increased in size, and I had lost hardly any fat!"
—Carol, Beloit, Wisconsin

WIDE ANGLE

Problem #2: Can't get motivated
Solution: Make a commitment.
- Read books, magazines, and newsletters for inspiration.
- Identify someone who's fit and use that person as a role model.
- Set specific, short-term goals. Reward yourself when you achieve them.
- Hang out with people who are interested in health and fitness.

Problem #3: Boredom
Solution: Make it interesting.
- Vary your exercise activities. Choose activities you really enjoy.
- Find an exercise partner and turn your exercise into a social occasion.
- Select different walking or biking paths for scenic variety.

Cross-Training
One of the best ways to stay motivated about exercise over the long haul is to cross-train. Alternating activities prevents boredom, prevents injuries, and works different muscles. It's the perfect way to enjoy different activities and stay in shape. Try alternating jogging with biking with your kids, playing tennis, or taking the dog for a long walk. Who said working out had to be boring?!

Perfect Exercises for Every Stage of Life

After reading this section of the book, you won't have any excuses not to make exercise an integral part of your everyday life no matter what stage of life you're in. Whether you're single, a young parent, or retired, we have exercises and tips for everyone.

Young Kids: Play, play, play. It's the best way for kids to get the exercise they need. Getting them involved in sports such as soccer, swimming, cross-country, skiing, basketball, lacrosse, or anything aerobic, is a great start to a lifetime of fitness.

Singles and Married with No Kids: This group of people tends to have more time to exercise. Work out with a partner or your spouse. This time can be spent sharing common interests and building your relationship. Learn a new sport. Train for an event like a running or biking race or a triathlon. Test yourself and push yourself beyond what you think are your limits. This time of your life is an ideal time to set the pattern for doing both aerobic exercise and strength training.

Married with Kids: This is such a busy time of life that you may wonder if there will ever be any time for yourself again. But don't give up on fitness just because Junior came along. Keep in mind:

- Buy a jogging stroller or one that can be pulled behind a bike, and take Junior along. There are even combination strollers out on the market that can be used for both running and biking.
- Alternate workout days with your spouse.
- Find a gym that provides baby-sitting.
- Trade baby-sitting with a neighbor so you can go work out.
- Join a community pool and go as a family. You and your spouse can switch watching the kids and swimming.
- Walk as much as you can. Get outside even when it's not so nice out.

Families with Older Kids: Since older kids have a more scheduled routine with school and after-school activities, you can plan your day better than when they were younger and you weren't quite sure when they would nap or sleep through the night. Because your days are becoming more routine, it doesn't mean they are any less busy. But make time for yourself. Get up early and workout. Do activities as a family. Play volleyball, touch football, jog, go to the pool, take bike rides, and hike. Making fitness a family affair sets a good example for your children. Keep in mind:

- Watch out, you weekend warriors. Injuries are high in people who are minimally active during the week and then go all-out on the weekend. Be sure to warm up adequately before exercise, and try and stay as active as possible during the week.
- Women need to be doing some form of weight-bearing aerobic exercise and/or strength training to help build bone and help prevent osteoporosis.

Retirement: Ahh, the kids are out of the house, and you have free time again. (Yeah, right. If you're actually one of those people who didn't take up another job or hobby or aren't involved in a million activities!) If you don't have any health or physical problems, the exercise field is wide open. Age is not a factor in whether you can walk, swim, jog, bike, do aerobics, cross-country ski, or lift weights. Train for a race. Prizes are often awarded to the winners of the sixty-five-and-over age group. Keep in mind:

- Be sure to see a doctor before starting any new exercises, especially if you have a history of heart problems in your family, or you have any knee or back pain.

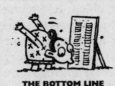

THE BOTTOM LINE

Fountain of Youth?

Research has shown no better way to slow or even reverse the progress of aging itself than through the combination of aerobic and strength-building exercise and a balanced, nutritious diet.

- Exercise is to the body what location is to real estate: the promise of a rewarding future. Who said people should take it easy as they age? Inactivity and bed rest for prolonged periods hasten the aging process and promote problems associated with the digestive and cardiovascular systems, bones, and muscles.
- By improving balance and mobility, strength and flexibility exercises may prevent falls and injuries. Falls are the leading cause of fatal injury in people over seventy-five.

Section 6
Cooking Healthy

Food Consciousness

Try this little exercise the next time you're sitting down to eat. Don't look at your food as something to fulfill your need for nourishment. Don't even desire it because of the way you know it'll taste. Look at it as a combination of very serious chemicals. Not chemicals that don't know how to take a joke. Rather, as chemicals that have their origin in other chemicals. Chemicals that come together in a marvelous fashion to make your food what it is.

Are you still hungry? Probably not. After all, who wants to eat chemicals?

But, really, God uses a variety of things to create the food you have. We want to raise your consciousness about two chemicals found in food that you might want to be aware of.

CHOLESTEROL

The American Heart Association (AHA) describes cholesterol as a soft, waxy substance found among the lipids (fats) in the bloodstream and in all your body's cells. Cholesterol is important because it's used to form cell membranes, some hormones, and other needed tissues. But a high level of cholesterol in the blood is a major risk factor for coronary heart disease, which causes heart attacks. Cholesterol and other fats can't dissolve in the blood. They have to be transported to and from the cells by special carriers of lipids and proteins called lipoproteins. Cholesterol is found in meat, poultry, seafood, and dairy products (egg yolks and organ meats have an especially high content). Cholesterol isn't found in fruits, vegetables, vegetable oils, grains, cereals, nuts, and seeds. Seafood varies in its cholesterol content.

So what's the word on cholesterol? It's simple, really. You need cholesterol for your body to function normally, but your body makes enough so that you don't need to get more from the foods you eat.

FATS

Fats are another important chemical to be conscious of as you're eating or preparing your food.

Saturated Fats

Saturated fatty acids are the main dietary culprit in raising blood cholesterol.

The AHA tells us that foods that contain saturated fats include beef, beef fat, veal, lamb, pork, lard, poultry fat, butter, cream, milk, cheeses, and other dairy products made from whole milk. Also, foods from plants that contain high amounts of saturated fatty acids include coconut oil, palm oil, and palm kernel oil (often called tropical oils) and cocoa butter.

Polyunsaturated Fats

Polyunsaturated fatty acids are often found in liquid oils of vegetable origin. They are also found in safflower, sesame, and sunflower seeds, corn and soybeans, and many nuts and seeds and their oils.

What's the big deal?

Really, it's about consciousness. Nope, not trying to become one with your food or even psychoanalyzing it. It's about looking at what you've got on your plate and asking the following questions:

- Will this food enhance or tear apart my diet?
- Will this food enhance my ability to be who I am?
- Will this food make me healthy?

If you can answer those questions positively, and with a clear conscience, then go ahead. . .chow down. But, if you aren't sure, or if you don't know what's in the food you eat, now is a great time to start researching.

We want you to discover two vital areas to being conscious of what's on your plate. First, we want to give you help with effective ways to eat out. Then, we'll give you some ideas for being more conscious with what you cook and eat at home.

EATING OUT

It's 6:35. Midweek church begins at 7:00. You just walked in from a long day at work. Before you is a banquet of decisions. Skip church and serve a healthy, well-balanced meal? Opt for fast-food and make it to church on time? The second option sounds great, but you're concerned about your kids getting enough healthy food. What should you do?

IS IT GOOD FOR YOU?

Well, it IS easier, but is eating out good for you?

Eating out *can* be good for you—just like eating at home *can* be good for you too. And eating out can be bad for you. Here are some things to watch for when you eat out.

WHERE TO EAT

If you drive around your town a lot, chances are you know the restaurant options that are before you. Most restaurants fall into one of the following classifications:

- **Fast-food:** These are restaurants that cater to those of us who either are, or live in, a hurry. And, while they're not always fast, we've grown used to their food. Fast-food restaurants fill the need of eating but sometimes lack the variety for choosing a healthy option.
- **Moderate joints:** These are restaurants that offer a higher price than the fast-food places, but you can still enjoy a meal in your shorts. They offer a wider variety than fast-food places.
- **Nice eateries:** Restaurants that fall into this category are places you might take someone for her birthday or to celebrate a promotion. The variety is balanced, the food is good, but the price might prohibit most of us from eating at these places regularly.
- **Save-up establishments:** If you save your pennies and have a super-duper moment you want to celebrate, you'd probably attend these places. They're expensive, the food is good, and the variety is often well thought out.

BEFORE YOU EAT

Believe it or not, there's a lot you can do before you even order your food at a restaurant. Here are some ideas from AHA's website found at: WWW.DELICIOUSDECISIONS.ORG/OA/EAT_BEFORE_MAIN.HTML.

- If you're familiar with the menu, decide what you'll order before you enter the restaurant. That will help you avoid the temptation of ordering something that will hurt you or your diet.
- If you're trying a new place, take some time to study the menu. This will help you avoid making split-second—and often regrettable—decisions.
- If your companions don't mind, remove unneeded temptations, such as butter, from the table.
- Drink two full glasses of water before eating your food.
- Avoid foods described in the following way: buttery, buttered, fried, pan-fried, creamed, escalloped, au gratin, or à la mode.

Ordering and Eating

You're ready to order. You're prepared to eat. What should you do? The AHA website continues with these helpful hints.

- Don't be shy. Ask about ingredients or preparation methods for the food you're not familiar with. You deserve to know what you're eating.
- Ask to substitute low-fat foods for high-fat ones. For example, ask for steamed vegetables in place of french fries or fresh fruit salad in place of mayonnaise-laden coleslaw.
- Ask the chef to remove the skin from poultry, or remove it yourself at the table.
- Order all dressings and sauces on the side, so you can control your portions. Use them sparingly or not at all.
- Ask to have your food prepared without butter or cream sauces.
- Order vegetable side dishes. Be sure to ask the server to leave off any sauces or butter.
- Be selective at salad bars and choose fresh greens, raw vegetables, fresh fruits, garbanzo beans, and low-fat dressing. Avoid cheeses, marinated salads, pasta salads, and fruit salads with whipped cream.
- Order foods that are steamed, broiled, grilled, stir-fried, or roasted. Or ask that your food be prepared with very little butter or oil or none at all.
- If you love potatoes, order them baked, boiled, or roasted—not fried. Ask to have the butter and sour cream left off. Try salsa or pepper and chives instead.
- For dessert, check your menu to see whether the restaurant offers low-fat dishes. If not, order fresh fruit or sorbet. Order fresh, seasonal fruit without whipped cream or a topping.

Eating at Home

SUBSTITUTING INGREDIENTS

When you were in grade school, you probably had a substitute. Remember what that was like? You probably got away with more. You might have even gotten a sub who loved to joke around. Well, substituting ingredients is a lot like that. Same situation, with something new making it interesting and lightening it up.

When you're cooking at home, replacing some of your favorite ingredients might not be the easiest thing in the world. Use the list

below to discover that replacing your favorite ingredients isn't as difficult as it sounds, and it might just be fun!

Here are some substitutes from www.gourmetconnection.com:

Sour cream: Plain low-fat yogurt or 1 cup cottage cheese blended with
1 1/2 teaspoon lemon juice, or fat-free sour cream

Whipped cream: Chilled, whipped, evaporated skim milk or a nondairy
whipped topping made from polyunsaturated fat

Cream: Evaporated skim milk

Whole milk: Skim, 1%, or 2% milk as a beverage or in recipes

Full-fat cheese: Low-fat, skim-milk cheese, cheese with less than five
grams of fat per ounce, or fat-free

Ricotta cheese: Low-fat or fat-free cottage cheese or nonfat or low-fat
ricotta cheese

Ice cream: Low-fat or nonfat ice cream or frozen low-fat or nonfat
yogurt, frozen fruit juice products, or sorbet

Ground beef: Extra lean ground beef or lean ground turkey or chicken

Bacon: Canadian bacon or lean ham

Sausage: Lean ground turkey or 95% fat-free sausage

Whole egg: Two egg whites or 1/4 cup cholesterol-free liquid egg product or one egg white plus two teaspoons oil

One egg yolk: One egg white

One egg (as thickener): One tablespoon flour

Mayonnaise: Low-fat or fat-free mayonnaise or whipped salad dressing
or plain low-fat yogurt combined with low-fat cottage cheese

Salad dressings: Low-calorie commercial dressings or homemade
dressing made with unsaturated oils, water, and vinegar or lemon
juice

Cream soups: Defatted broths or broth-based or skim-milk-based
soups

Nuts: Dried fruit, such as raisins, chopped dried apricots, or
dried cranberries.

One-ounce baking chocolate: Three tablespoons cocoa powder and
one tablespoon oil

Butter, lard, and other saturated fats (coconut oil, palm oil): Soft,
tub margarine (first ingredient on food label as liquid vegetable oil);
corn, cottonseed, olive, rapeseed (canola), safflower, sesame, soy-
bean, or sunflower oil

Healthy Recipes

You're ready to leap into a healthier you. You're prepared for the challenge of fixing new foods and trying new things. Here are a few plain old healthy recipes to get you started.

Spicy Spaghetti with Beef & Vegetables
Ingredients
1 pkg (7 ozs) uncooked spaghetti
1/2 lb lean ground beef, crumbled
1/4 cup chopped onion
1 can (15 ozs) tomato sauce
1 tablespoon red wine vinegar
1 teaspoon Italian seasoning
1/2 teaspoon sugar
1/4 teaspoon garlic powder
1/4 teaspoon crushed red pepper flakes
1 medium zucchini, thinly sliced (1 cup)
1 medium tomato, seeded and coarsely chopped (1 cup)
2 tablespoons to 1/4 cup snipped fresh parsley
Directions
Prepare spaghetti as directed on package. Rinse in hot water. Drain. Set aside.

Combine beef and onion in 10-inch nonstick skillet. Cook over medium heat for 4 to 5 minutes, or until meat is no longer pink, stirring occasionally. Stir in tomato sauce, vinegar, Italian seasoning, sugar, garlic powder, and red pepper flakes. Cook over medium heat for 2 to 4 minutes or until hot and bubbly, stirring occasionally. Stir in prepared spaghetti and zucchini. Cook for 2 to 3 minutes or until hot, stirring occasionally. Stir in tomato and parsley. Serve hot.

Yields 6 servings.

Black-Bean Chili
Ingredients
4 cans (15 ozs each) black beans, rinsed and drained, divided
1 can (14 1/2 ozs) ready-to-serve chicken broth
1 small onion, chopped (1/2 cup)
1 stalk celery, thinly sliced (1/2 cup)
1/3 cup chopped green pepper
2 cloves garlic, minced

2 teaspoons olive oil
1 can (14 1/2 ozs) whole tomatoes, undrained and cut up
2 teaspoons chili powder
1/2 teaspoon ground cumin
1/2 teaspoon dried oregano leaves
1/4 teaspoon salt
1/2 cup chopped seeded tomato
1/2 cup sliced green onions
2 tablespoons plus 2 teaspoons plain nonfat or low-fat yogurt

Directions

Place 3 cups beans and the broth in food processor or blender. Process until smooth. Combine onion, celery, pepper, garlic and oil in 3-quart saucepan. Cook over medium heat for 8 to 10 minutes or until vegetables are tender, stirring frequently. Add processed beans, remaining beans, the canned tomatoes, chili powder, cumin, oregano, and salt. Mix well. Bring to boil over high heat, stirring occasionally. Reduce heat to low. Cook for 10 to 15 minutes, or until chili is hot and flavors are blended, stirring occasionally. Garnish each serving with 1 tablespoon each chopped tomato and green onion and 1 teaspoon yogurt.

Yields 8 servings.

South of the Border Muffuletta

Ingredients

1 loaf (1 lb) round sourdough bread
1/4 cup nonfat yogurt cheese
1 tablespoon sliced green onion
1 clove garlic, minced
1 teaspoon Dijon mustard
1/8 teaspoon chili powder
1/8 teaspoon ground cumin
1/8 teaspoon ground turmeric
6 slices (1/2 oz each) fully cooked chicken breast
3 slices (1 oz each) reduced-fat Monterey Jack cheese
1 can (4 ozs) whole green chilies, drained and sliced in half lengthwise
4 slices tomato
Leaf lettuce

Directions

Cut loaf in half crosswise. Cut circle 1 inch from outer edge of crust. Remove bread from circle to 1-inch depth. Reserve bread for future use. Set halves aside. Combine yogurt cheese, onion, garlic, mustard, chili

powder, cumin, and turmeric in small mixing bowl. Spread evenly over inside of top and bottom halves of loaf. Layer 2 chicken slices, half of chilies, 2 tomato slices, and lettuce on bottom half of loaf. Repeat layers once. Top with 2 chicken slices and 1 cheese slice.
Place top half of loaf over filling. Serve in wedges.

    Yields 6 servings.

Tomato-Basil Soup
Ingredients
1/2 cup chopped shallots
1 clove garlic, minced
1 teaspoon olive oil
1 can (28 ozs) Roma tomatoes, undrained and cut up
1/2 cup water
1/4 teaspoon snipped fresh basil leaves
1/2 teaspoon instant chicken bouillon granules
1/2 teaspoon sugar
1/2 teaspoon freshly ground pepper
4 fresh Roma tomatoes, chopped (2 cups), divided
1 cup skim milk, divided
Directions
Combine shallots, garlic, and oil in 2-quart saucepan. Cook over medium heat for 3 to 3 1/2 minutes or until tender, stirring frequently. Add canned tomatoes, water, basil, bouillon, sugar, and pepper. Cook for 5 1/2 to 8 minutes or until mixture is hot and flavors are blended, stirring occasionally. Remove from heat. Combine half of tomato mixture, 2 Roma tomatoes, and 1/2 cup milk in food processor or blender. Process until smooth. Set purée aside. Repeat with remaining ingredients. Return purée to saucepan. Cook over medium heat for 8 to 10 minutes or until soup is hot, stirring occasionally. Spoon into serving dishes. Top each serving with crostini*, if desired.
* To make crostini, arrange 6 slices of toasted Italian bread on baking sheet. Brush slices evenly with 1 tablespoon olive oil. Top each with 2 thin slices fresh Roma tomato, 1 small fresh basil leaf, and 1 tablespoon shredded fresh Parmesan cheese. Broil 5 inches from heat for 4 or 5 minutes, or until golden brown.

    Yields 6 servings.

Baked Spinach Fettuccini
Ingredients

1 pkg (9 ozs) fresh spinach fettuccini, cut into quarters; or 8 oz dry
   spinach fettuccini, broken in half
1/4 cup unseasoned dry bread crumbs, divided
1 cup frozen cholesterol-free egg product, defrosted; or 4 eggs, beaten
1 cup chopped red pepper
1 small onion
1/2 cup low-fat or nonfat ricotta cheese
1/4 cup shredded fresh Parmesan cheese
1 tablespoon olive oil
2 teaspoons Italian seasoning
2 cloves garlic, minced
3/4 teaspoon salt
1/4 teaspoon white pepper

Directions

Heat oven to 375 degrees. Prepare pasta as directed on package. Drain.
Set aside. Spray 9-inch round baking dish with nonstick vegetable cooking spray. Sprinkle inside of dish with 2 tablespoons bread crumbs, tilt-
ing dish to coat sides. Repeat with nonstick vegetable cooking spray
and remaining 2 tablespoons bread crumbs. Set crust aside. Combine
remaining ingredients, except pasta, in large mixing bowl. Add pasta to
pepper mixture and stir together. Slide pasta mixture evenly into prepared dish. Spray piece of foil with nonstick vegetable cooking spray.
Cover dish with foil. Bake for 45 to 50 minutes, or until crust is deep
golden brown. Remove foil. Bake for an additional 10 to 15 minutes or
until knife inserted in center comes out clean. (Surface may appear
slightly moist.) Loosen sides of fettuccini with spatula or knife. Invert
dish onto serving plate. (Do not remove dish.) Let stand for 10 minutes.
Gently remove dish. Serve fettuccini in wedges. Serve with hot, low-fat
pasta sauce, if desired.

　　　Yields 6 servings.

Pineapple Carrot Cake
Ingredients
Cake

1/2 cup all-purpose flour
1/2 cup whole wheat flour
1/2 cup packed brown sugar
1 teaspoon pumpkin pie spice

1 teaspoon baking powder
1/2 teaspoon baking soda
1 can (8 ozs) crushed pineapple in juice, drained (reserve 3 tablespoons
        juice for topping)
1/2 cup frozen cholesterol-free egg product, defrosted; or 2 eggs
1/4 cup vegetable oil
1 cup shredded carrots
1/2 cup raisins (optional)

Topping
4 ozs light or nonfat cream cheese, softened
1/3 cup powdered sugar
1/4 teaspoon pumpkin pie spice

Directions
Heat oven to 350 degrees. Spray 9-inch round cake pan with nonstick
vegetable cooking spray. Dust lightly with all-purpose flour. Set aside.
Combine all cake ingredients except carrots and raisins in large mixing
bowl. Beat at low speed of electric mixer just until combined. Beat at
high speed for 2 minutes, scraping bowl frequently. Fold in carrots and
raisins. Pour batter into prepared pan. Bake for 20 to 25 minutes or
until wooden toothpick inserted in center comes out clean. Remove
cake from pan. Place on serving plate. In small mixing bowl, combine
all topping ingredients and reserved juice. Beat at medium speed of
electric mixer until smooth. Spread topping on cooled cake. Sprinkle
with additional shredded carrot, if desired.

   Microwave tip: Microwave prepared topping on high for 30 to 45
seconds or until warm, stirring once. Spoon warm topping over wedges
of warm cake.

   Yields 6 servings.

[ABOVE RECIPES FROM WWW.HEALTHYCHOICE.COM]

Dream Recipes Tailored for Your Diet
We know that we've suggested a lot of information in this book. And,
just so you know that we're serious about what we're asking, we've
included a few recipes for each of the diets that we've discussed in this
book. Feel free to use, adapt, and change these to fit your lifestyle.

PROTEIN DIET RECIPES

Cuban Turkey Picadillo
Ingredients
2 lbs boneless turkey, diced finely or ground
2 teaspoons ground cumin
2 teaspoons garlic powder
4 tablespoons ketchup
2 chicken bouillon cubes
2 tablespoons olive oil
1/2 medium onion, diced
1/2 medium bell pepper, diced
4 ozs stuffed green olives, diced well
4 tablespoons capers plus 2 tablespoons caper brine
1/2 teaspoon black pepper
2 tablespoons wheat bran
Directions
Combine turkey, black pepper, garlic powder, and cumin in a bowl. Let set for 10 minutes. Fry the onion and bell pepper in the oil over medium-high heat until the onions are clear. Add the turkey mixture and cook until the turkey begins to cook well. Add the remaining ingredients except the bran; cover and bring to a boil. Reduce heat and let simmer about 20 minutes. Remove from the heat and stir in the bran. Let set 10 minutes before serving.

Yields 4 servings.

Italian Beef a la Covelli
Ingredients
2 lbs stew beef
1 1/2 cups water
1/2 medium onion, diced
2 teaspoons Italian seasoning
2 bouillon cubes
1 whole bay leaf
2 teaspoons garlic powder
2 tablespoons wheat bran
Directions
Place the onions, seasonings, and bouillon cubes in a large pan. Place the beef in the pan. Add the liquids. Cover and bring to a boil. Reduce heat and simmer about an hour and a half, stirring every 15 minutes.

Remove from heat; remove the bay leaf and add the bran. Stir again. Let sit at least 15 minutes before serving. Serve with a half cup of au jus.

Yields about 4 servings.

Pepperoni Chicken
Ingredients
2 lbs boneless chicken, cut into 1/2-inch cubes
2 teaspoons olive oil
1/4 lb pepperoni, sliced
1/2 bell pepper, diced
4 ozs black olives
2 teaspoons garlic powder
1 teaspoon anise or fennel
2 bouillon cubes
1/2 teaspoon pepper
1 cup shredded mozzarella cheese
1/2 cup Parmesan cheese
1 tablespoon wheat bran

Directions
In an ovenproof skillet, fry the chicken in the oil over medium-high heat until it begins to brown slightly. Add the onions and cook until they begin to clear. Add the remaining ingredients except the bran, pepperoni, and cheese; cover and bring to a boil. Reduce heat and simmer 45 minutes. After 45 minutes, turn on the oven broiler. Remove the lid and stir in the pepperoni and bran. Sprinkle the Parmesan cheese over the contents of the skillet, then the mozzarella, and put under the broiler until the cheese browns.

Yields 4 servings.

COUNTING CALORIES RECIPES

Grilled Steak and Vegetable Salad
A delicious salad and entrée all in one, creating a light main course that's a great change of pace.

Ingredients

1 1/2 pounds beef flank steak, fat trimmed, scored
6 medium Italian plum tomatoes, cut into wedges
1 medium green pepper, sliced
1 medium sweet onion, cut into small wedges
4 ears corn, cooked, cut into 1 1/2-inch pieces
Fresh Herb Vinaigrette (recipe follows)

Directions

Grill steak over medium-hot coals to desired degree of doneness, about 20 minutes for medium, turning steak halfway through cooking time. Slice steak diagonally across grain into scant 1/4-inch slices.

Combine sliced meat and vegetables in shallow serving bowl. Pour dressing over and toss. Serve immediately or refrigerate several hours and serve chilled.

Note: If desired, steak can be broiled rather than grilled for the same amount of time.

Yields 6 servings.

Fresh Herb Vinaigrette
Ingredients

1/3 cup red wine vinegar
3 tablespoons olive or vegetable oil
2 cloves garlic, minced
3 tablespoons minced fresh or 1 teaspoon dried rosemary leaves
3 tablespoons minced fresh or 1 teaspoon dried oregano leaves
1/2 teaspoon salt
1/4 cup water
2 tablespoons fresh lemon juice
2 tablespoons NutraSweet Spoonful
3 tablespoons minced fresh or 1/2 teaspoon dried thyme leaves
3 tablespoons minced fresh or 1 teaspoon dried basil leaves
1/4 teaspoon pepper

Directions

Combine all ingredients in covered jar; shake to mix.

Yields 3/4 cup.

Patriotic Cheesecake

A "light is right" patriotic salute to cheesecake, decked out with blueberry and raspberry stars and stripes.

Ingredients

3 cups vanilla wafer crumbs
3 tablespoons NutraSweet Spoonful
1 cup skim milk
1 pkg (3 oz) reduced-fat cream cheese, softened
1 tablespoon grated lemon rind
1/3 to 1/2 cup NutraSweet Spoonful
2 pints raspberries
4 tablespoons margarine, melted
1 envelope (1/4 oz) unflavored gelatin
2 pkgs (8 ozs each) reduced-fat cream cheese, softened
2 tablespoons lemon juice
2 teaspoons vanilla
1 pint blueberries

Directions

Mix crumbs, margarine, and 3 tablespoons Nutrasweet Spoonful in medium bowl; pat evenly on bottom of jelly roll pan, 15 x 10 inches. Sprinkle gelatin over milk in small saucepan; let stand 2 to 3 minutes. Heat over medium-low heat, stirring constantly, until gelatin is dissolved. Cool to room temperature. Beat cream cheese until fluffy in large bowl; gradually beat in milk mixture. Beat in lemon juice and rind, vanilla and 1/3 to 1/2 cup NutraSweet Spoonful. Pour mixture over crust; refrigerate until set, 3 to 4 hours. Before serving, decorate to look like a flag, using the blueberries for the stars, the raspberries for the stripes.

Yields 16 servings.

[SOURCE FOR LOW-CAL RECIPES: WWW.CALORIECONTROL.ORG]

Low-Fat Recipes

Better-Built Burger
Ingredients
1 1/2 pounds ground turkey breast
1/2 cup finely chopped onion
1 tablespoon Worcestershire sauce
6 whole-grain buns
Topping
3/4 cup toppings of choice: sliced onion, tomato, cucumber, sprouts,
lettuce, honey mustard (2 teaspoons) or barbecue sauce (2 teaspoons)
Directions
Combine ground turkey breast, onion, and Worcestershire sauce in a
large bowl. Mix well. Divide turkey mixture into 6 equal portions. Place
burger into nonstick pan. Cover and "fry" burger over moderate heat
until golden brown and cooked through and white inside. Toast buns.
Put burger on bun — add toppings of choice.
     Yields 6 servings.

Bananas "Foster"
Ingredients
3 firm bananas
3 tablespoons dark brown sugar
1 tablespoon butter
Cardamom or cinnamon to taste
1/2 cup half-and-half
Directions
Preheat oven to 450 degrees. Peel and slice the bananas into a baking
dish. Crumble the brown sugar over the bananas. Bake 5 minutes.
Dot with butter. Divide equally onto dessert plates. Sprinkle with
cardamom or cinnamon. Pour half-and-half around the bananas and
serve immediately.
Note: Instead of frying the bananas in butter, this recipe bakes them
instead. Serving them with half-and-half instead of ice cream also saves
fat and calories.
     Yields 4 servings.

[TWO ABOVE LOW-FAT RECIPES FROM HTTP://CI.SHREWSBURY.MA.US/SPS/SCHOOLS/HIGH/DEPT/HLTH/FATS/LOWFAT.HTML]

Chicken Picatta
Ingredients

1 lb boneless, skinless chicken breast, sliced thin for scallopini—be sure to trim the fat!

2 to 4 cloves garlic, pressed or minced fine

1 large shallot, minced fine

1 cup defatted chicken stock

Juice of 1 lemon

Basil, oregano, and pepper to taste

Flour for dusting

1 to 2 teaspoons olive oil

1 tablespoon capers (optional)

1 cup dry white wine

Directions

Dust chicken pieces until well coated. Heat 1 teaspoon oil on high and lightly brown chicken on both sides. Do not overcook. Remove and set aside. Lower heat to medium. Add remaining oil and sauté garlic and shallot until translucent. Add seasonings and chicken. Turn up heat to high and add wine. Boil off alcohol, and add stock and lemon juice. Reduce until slightly thickened. Add capers if desired and serve.

Asian Grilled Chicken Salad
Ingredients

2 chicken breasts, split in half

4 cups fresh assorted greens, Bibb lettuce, Frieze, spinach, Red Leaf lettuce, etc.

1 cucumber, split in half, seeded and sliced in matchsticks

1 carrot, shredded

1 to 2 green onions, thinly sliced

1/2 pkg Raman noodles, uncooked, broken into small pieces

2 mandarin oranges or 1 small tangerine, peeled, broken into sections

Five-spice powder, salt, and pepper to taste (optional)

Five-spice Powder

5 teaspoons ground anise (aniseed)

5 teaspoons star anise

1 cinnamon stick (5 inches) in cassia bark

2 tablespoons whole cloves

7 teaspoons fennel seeds

Directions
Using a blender, process all ingredients until finely ground. Store in an airtight jar up to three months.

Dressing
1/2 cup light soy sauce—preferably low sodium
2 tablespoons rice wine vinegar
3 tablespoons defatted chicken broth
1 clove garlic, pressed or finely chopped
1 teaspoon fresh ginger, pressed or grated
1 pinch of sugar
1/2 to 1 teaspoon toasted sesame oil

Directions
In a small bowl combine soy sauce, vinegar, broth, and sugar. Whisk well until sugar is dissolved. Add garlic and ginger and mix well. Add oil and whisk until well blended. Set aside. Season chicken if desired and grill for 3 to 5 minutes on each side or until cooked through. This will go quickly since the chicken breast pieces are very thin. Set aside. In a large bowl, combine greens and add cucumber, carrots, and green onion. Whisk dressing again and drizzle over salad. Toss well so that the salad is well coated. Arrange salad on plate. Slice chicken on the diagonal and arrange artfully on the salad. Top with noodle pieces and garnish with orange sections. Serve immediately.

[ABOVE TWO RECIPES FROM HTTP://WWW.LIGHTLIVING.COM/MRARCHIVE.HTML]

Section 7
....
Attitudes
Toward Food

More Than a Swoosh

Lindsey has always loved the trapeze. And, in this moment, everything she's loved and trained for have come together. Years of training all fall on the shoulders of this one moment. Hands dusted with chalk. Hair neatly tied back. A little too much stage makeup.

Swoosh. Swoosh. Swoosh.

Lindsey swung back and forth under the big top. On the other side, Raymond was doing likewise. Arms outstretched and waiting to catch her. All she had to do now was repeat everything she'd been practicing for months.

Swoosh. Swoosh. Swoosh.

"Alright, I'll just let go; do a couple of flips. Raymond will catch me. And later, we'll celebrate with a low-fat latte. Just gotta get through this. Why am I so scared?" The "what-ifs" began to creep up Lindsey's back. "What if Raymond doesn't catch me? What if that net *doesn't* hold?"

Swoosh. Swoosh. Swoosh.

Raymond began to wonder if Lindsey would ever let go. He stopped counting her swings around the twenty-fifth swoosh. "Come on, Lindsey! I'll catch you. Let's get this thing going!"

Swoosh. Swoosh. Swoosh.

Hours later, firemen came and helped Lindsey down from the trapeze. Lindsey never completed the trick. Even though she was trained, well practiced, and trusted the safety net, she couldn't get over the fear of what might happen.

Imagine, having all of the information and training and still not being able to complete the one task you've been working for your whole life. What a tragedy.

Our attitude toward food confronts us with the same reality. There's tons of information out about healthy eating. There are more than enough diet plans to choose from. But our fear of what might, or might not happen, keeps many of us from taking that first step. That fear prevents us from saying no to our favorite calorie-filled dessert or helps us indulge in something we know might hurt us, hoping to possibly fill a deeper need.

In this chapter we want to discuss some ways to look at food differently, how the Bible presents food, and we'll look at one of the most influential diet options around today—the Weigh Down Diet.

GETTING PERSPECTIVE

Before we begin discussing how to think rightly about food, we'd like you to write down some of your ideas about food. Get a handle on your view of food by answering the following:

• What does food do?

_____

_____

• Give three reasons why we need food.

_____

_____

_____

_____

Now, before you read on, read back over what you've just written. Do you agree with all of your responses? If you want to change anything, now's the time to do it. Great. Let's move on.

Thinking rightly about food is totally about perspective. It's about noticing the value that food has, but it's also about realizing the effects and the damage that food can do to you. We want to help you get that perspective.

WHAT GOD CREATED

Later on you'll see that God created food for us. In fact, He created food for us to not only crave (for nourishment), but He also created food with a texture, smell, and appearance. He created us to like food; that's how He put us together. He made us to not only *need* food; He put things in us that would cause us to *enjoy* food.

Taste Buds
If you'll look at the front and back of your tongue, you'll notice little dots.

And (as everyone older than the age of four knows), those dots are taste buds. God created each food with a particular taste. And He made those little tiny sensors so we'd be able to enjoy what He created. God thought ahead. He prepared us for the wonderful tastes He worked hard to form.

Stomach

Churning more efficiently than a bread maker, and more powerfully than many model planes is the stomach. If God's work on the taste bud doesn't wow you, consider God's work on the stomach. Once you eat, food passes down your esophagus and lands in your stomach. There, the stomach churns the food around, breaking it down and absorbing nutrients into the wall of the stomach. And from there, the nutrients are carried off to the rest of the body.

Appearance

What gets your mouth watering? Chances are, it's the way your favorite food looks. Sure, you remember the way it tastes, but the way it looks is probably just as appealing.

God didn't just do His best work on us; He worked hard on creating things that He knew we would find visually appealing. Fruit. Vegetables. Hamburgers. Okay, God didn't exactly create hamburgers, but you get the point.

Smell

Describe the way that bread smells. Paint a picture of the smell that brownies have fresh out of the oven. Whatever you describe or paint might just be considered an overwhelming story or modern-day work of art.

That's because one of the most powerful senses is smell. It's something God uses to draw us to the foods we enjoy. In fact, once we smell something we love to eat, our stomach begins to produce the enzymes needed to digest the food. We don't even have to taste it for our body to go into action.

Those four factors draw us into the process of eating. And, in fact, we need all of these in order to eat and enjoy our food. Ask anyone who has lost his sense of smell, and he'll tell you that he enjoys his food less. Discuss eating with someone who has difficulty digesting foods, and she's sure to tell you that eating is less enjoyable.

We need to be able to see, smell, taste, and digest our food. And that's the way that God created us. To eat. And, in eating, our bodies receive the nourishment we need in order to live.

KNOW THE DIFFERENCE

All of these really cool things come together to make eating an enjoyable moment for most of us. We need food. We enjoy food. But often our enjoyment merges with our need and the two get blurred. We end up eating when we really don't need to, or we eat the wrong foods.

Beginning the process of thinking rightly about the food you eat means understanding the difference between desire and hunger.

Desire

This is something your mind creates when it gets to attached to the food you like. Desire sets in when you feel lonely. Or when you lose control over your ability to say no to your favorite food. Desire is tricky. It can make you think you're hungry, when what's really happening is that you're craving a taste, texture, or smell.

Hunger

When your body needs food, or when your body is missing a vital nutrient, it signals your brain that it's time to eat. It even gives your brain clues as to what type of food you'll need. If you're craving salt, chances are you're lacking sodium.

Hunger is what God put in us to remind us to eat. But that internal clock can get confused with desire. When it does, our eating can go way off track.

THREE QUESTIONS

So those two factors decide what and when you'll eat. Listen to your mind (your desires), which sometimes thinks you're hungry, and you'll eat certain stuff at certain times. Listen to your stomach (your body), which knows when you really are hungry, and you'll eat different stuff at different times.

Overall, though, the goal is to strive to be ruled by your stomach. Eat only when you're hungry—not when you smell that pizza, see the burger, or get a craving for something sweet.

Help yourself evaluate what you put into your body by asking three simple questions before you eat anything.

- **What am I eating?**
  Are you about to put something in your mouth that will harm your body? Is the food you're about to eat something your body really needs or will it be turned mostly into waste?

- *Why am I eating?*
  Will what you're about to eat fill your need for nourishment? Or are you eating because you saw something you just couldn't resist?

- *When am I eating?*
  Regularity is the key to success in proclaiming your power over food. Are you about to eat something very late at night? Are you about to chow down on your third in-between meal snack?

Busting through the Mental Challenges

Your attitude about food comes down to a war between your willpower and your mind. It's a mental game. And, like it or not, this is a game you have to win. Consider trying these strategies for winning this important battle.

- *Prioritize*
  Begin asking yourself how important food is to you. Look for areas in which food needs to take a backseat to other desires, like worshipping God or serving unbelievers.

- *Learn your body*
  Learn the signals your body sends when it's hungry. Learn the signals it sends when it's just experiencing an empty craving. Get to know your body so well that you're ready with the proper response, no matter what the signal is.

- *Make advance decisions*
  No doubt, you'll be confronted with opportunities to eat food that won't do you a bit of good. Spend some time writing out your response to people who offer you tempting (but diet-breaking) foods. If you plan before you're tempted, you'll likely steer clear of giving in.

God Speaks on Food

God has a lot to say about food. And what He says is recorded in His Word. When you read God's views about food, it becomes very clear that God has some particular themes He wants to get across. Following are four principles that God makes crystal clear in His Word.

Provision

Since Creation, God has been demonstrating His love for us through providing. For many of us, that theme works its way into all facets of our lives. God has provided places to live, a life partner, children, etc. But, at its very basic element, God's provision is very simple. God loves us, and He longs to provide for us. God's provision for us in the area of food places immediate perspective on the food we eat.

What does God's Word say about His power to provide? Look at these passages.

"Then God said,'I give you every seed-bearing plant on the face of the whole earth and every tree that has fruit with seed in it. They will be yours for food' " (Genesis 1:29).

"The fear and dread of you will fall upon all the beasts of the earth and all the birds of the air, upon every creature that moves along the ground, and upon all the fish of the sea; they are given into your hands. Everything that lives and moves will be food for you. Just as I gave you the green plants, I now give you everything" (Genesis 9:2–3).

God's principle of provision leads us to a life of thankfulness. But it also ought to lead to a reverence for what we put into our bodies. God didn't just create us; He created the substance that causes us to grow.

Perspective

In Paul's day, the Jews had a problem. They loved their religious regulations—especially the ones about food. They gloried in what they ate. And, in being so concerned about what they put into their bodies, their stomachs became more important to them than God. They lost focus. They lost perspective.

A second principle to keep in mind is to focus on God first, and let God lead you to foods that will enhance who you are. The flip side of this principle is pointed out in this passage.

"Join with others in following my example, brothers, and take note of those who live according to the pattern we gave you. For, as I have often told you before and now say again even with tears, many live as enemies of the cross of Christ. Their destiny is destruction, their god is their stomach, and their glory is in their shame. Their mind is on earthly things. But our citizenship is in heaven. And we eagerly await a Savior from there, the Lord Jesus Christ, who, by the power that enables him to bring everything under his control, will transform our lowly bodies so that they will be like his glorious body" (Philippians 3:17–21).

Portions
The people in Amos's day had a big problem. They loved what they had, but they had too much of it. They ended up laying around, eating way too much, and getting overweight.

This principle is about more than how much food we put on our plate; it's also about being lazy. God wants eating to be a part of our day, not take over our entire day. And He wants us to go out and work, fellowship, and serve others. And we can't do that if we're lying around eating candy.

Check out what the people in Amos's time were doing.

"You lie on beds inlaid with ivory and lounge on your couches. You dine on choice lambs and fattened calves. You strum away on your harps like David and improvise on musical instruments. You drink wine by the bowlful and use the finest lotions, but you do not grieve over the ruin of Joseph. Therefore you will be among the first to go into exile; your feasting and lounging will end" (Amos 6:4–7).

Praise
The final principle that we want to highlight is the principle of praise. Everything we have comes from God. Everything we are is because of who He is. God's creative power demands our response. It's not as simple as uttering a "Praise God!" as we head off for work in the mornings. It means living a lifestyle that praises God by honoring what we have.

And beyond that, God desires that we do everything in response to who He is. We're to do everything to the glory of God, because He's the only One who deserves it.

God's Word is full of passages that describe our attitude of living a life of praise. Here are two:

"So whether you eat or drink or whatever you do, do it all for the glory of God" (1 Corinthians 10:31).

"And whatever you do, whether in word or deed, do it all in the name of the Lord Jesus, giving thanks to God the Father through him" (Colossians 3:17).

Weighing Down with Weigh Down

If there's any diet scheme that has properly married the concepts of proper perspective on food and biblical principles, it's the Weigh Down Diet created by Gwen Shamblin.

Shamblin used to be an overeater. For years she was thin because her exercise level was exactly equal to her overeating tendencies. However, as she grew older, her appetite grew and food got the best of her. After years of dieting, trying endless ways to lose the weight, she began copying the eating habits of a skinny friend. She decided to eat anything she wanted, but only when she was hungry. The result? Shamblin lost all her excess weight. And she's maintained her weight.

But her drive for discovering dieting principles didn't end there. After realizing that she was learning something that was not a part of other diets, she began to pray about what God might have her do with all of the information she had gained. It was at this point that God used Shamblin to begin the Weigh Down Diet.

THE WEIGH DOWN FOCUS

What's most unusual about this eating plan is that it doesn't want you to focus on what you're eating, and it even encourages you to stop dieting. What it *does* do is ask you to focus yourself and your efforts toward God. As you're revising the way you eat, Shamblin asks participants to seek God's approval for who they are and what they're eating. When participants begin feeling like a failure, Shamblin points them heavenward and encourages them to seek God's direction for whether they're really failing. In short, this diet urges you to focus yourself completely on God.

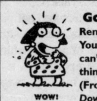

Good Point
Remember this: Your stomach can't taste anything!
(From the *Weigh Down Workshop*, page 110).

WOW!

THE TWO HOLES THEORY

Every one of us has been created with two holes that need to be filled. One is our stomachs, which need to be filled with food when we're hungry. The other empty place is our hearts. However, many of us try and fill the empty places in our hearts with food. Shamblin helps Weigh Down participants seek acceptance from God and pursue a relationship with God to fill the voids in their hearts.

THE BASIC PREMISE

The Weigh Down Diet is based on technical ideas, clinical research, and dieting principles. But the basic concept is fairly simple. When you're full, stop eating. That means, if you're in the middle of your favorite hamburger and you feel full, stop!

Shamblin encourages participants to recognize when they're "politely full," which is something described as full, but still being able to pick up your napkin without losing your meal. And the best advice available for recognizing when you're full is to slow down. Eating slowly can help you recognize when you're full much sooner than if you're eating quickly.

THE BENEFITS

Reading through *The Weigh Down Diet* book will give you clear indications that this diet is replete with benefits. It offers a total way of life. It provides a way for balance without prescribing a certain set of beliefs.

THE DISADVANTAGES

As with any system or philosophy, the Weigh Down Diet has its disadvantages. You won't find heavily prescribed dieting plans. You won't find recipes. That's because this diet is more about your relationship with God and getting perspective than it is about giving you rules and strict guidelines to follow.

More Info

If you want to check out this diet, consider the following options.

- You can buy *The Weigh Down Diet* book by Gwen Shamblin. It's published by Doubleday.
- You can surf their web page at http://www.wdworkshop.com.
- When you surf their web page, you can find out more information on an upcoming Weigh Down Workshop coming to your area.
- Subscribe to their magazine, *Exodus*, by calling 1-800-844-5208.

Eating Disorders

"I am sooo fat."

"I'm going to have to run five miles to work off this hamburger."

Common statements we've all heard before, but they could be a sign of deeper problems. Eating disorders are becoming more prevalent in our society every year, but the specific cause still baffles doctors and clinicians. Some speculate the cause is from society's pressure to be thin. Others say there are neurological links to depression and impulsive behavior, while others claim it's an inability to cope with problems. But they all agree that people battling eating disorders need multifaceted treatment that includes both nutritional and psychological counseling.

ANOREXIA

Jill is a superachiever in school and maintains a hectic schedule with activities at school, church, and in the community. She is pretty but is not satisfied with her weight. At 5 feet 7 inches tall, Jill weighs eighty-seven pounds and is determined to lose more. The epitome of self-discipline, she watches her diet with an eagle eye, avoiding carbohydrates and fats like they have the plague and eating only small amounts of lean meats and vegetables. If she feels like she's gained an ounce of weight, Jill exercises excessively to work it off. Undernourished, she has

---

WIDE ANGLE

Ask Yourself

Getting a handle on these three questions can take some time. But if you'll commit them to memory now, asking them every time you eat something becomes more feasible. Begin asking them now. Below each question, write out how you're doing in each area.

• What am I eating?

_____

• Do I regularly eat foods that help or hurt my body?

_____

• Why am I eating?

_____

• Do I tend to eat out of a sense of spontaneity?

_____

• When am I eating?

_____

• Am I prone to eat late at night or between meals often?

_____

stopped menstruating and become moody. She insists she's too fat, and when she looks in the mirror she sees a distorted view of herself. Despite her pencil-thin body, she determines to exercise even more and eat even less, when someone tells her she looks good. Jill has anorexia nervosa.

Why Do People Develop Anorexia?

The people with anorexia are mostly white females (although it does affect some males), from middle- or upper-middle-class families. Feeling the need to be perfect and often living up to expectations and ideals set by others, especially their parents, these girls lack their own identity. Although they may not feel controlled by others, they sense a lack of control over their own life. Controlling their eating is one way they gain control over their own lives. Other girls find themselves unable to deal with past or current problems, and controlling their body redirects their focus away from painful issues. There are many complex reasons why people develop anorexia. But because anorexia is shrouded in denial, it is difficult to pinpoint one specific cause. The physical consequences, however, are always the same.

Common Factors among People with Anorexia

THE BOTTOM LINE

1. Desire control
2. Strive for perfection
3. Value achievement and outward appearance more than inner sense of self worth
4. Often children of alcoholics or abusive parents

Physical Consequences to Anorexia

Essentially, anorexia is a form of self-starvation, so the extreme effects are similar to those seen in starving people in third-world countries—deep hollows in the face, major loss of muscle and fat mass, and visible bones. Other consequences include:
- Extreme weight loss
- Low blood pressure
- Weakened, inefficient heart
- Vitamin and mineral deficiencies
- Increase of fine body hair
- Skin dryness
- Decreased skin and core temperatures

- Sleep disturbances and bad dreams
- Fatigue
- Amenorrhea (loss of menstruation)
- Digestive tract unable to absorb nutrients
- Diarrhea

Diagnosis of Anorexia

Because everyone is in some pursuit of thinness (if you weren't, you wouldn't be reading this book), anorexia is sometimes difficult to diagnose. Anorexia-like thought patterns are common among many women, especially fashion models, dancers, gymnasts, and long-distance runners. Many people at some point or another exhibit one or more of the patterns, so it takes a skilled technician to make a diagnosis. But there are some basic tendencies that people with anorexia exhibit. If you know someone who is gradually losing more and more weight and looking "too thin" or unhealthy, she might have a problem with anorexia. Ask yourself the following questions:

1. Is her body weight below the normal minimal weight for her age and height?
2. Does she have an intense fear of gaining weight or becoming fat even though visibly thin?
3. Does she view herself as being fat or claim to "feel fat" even though underweight?
4. Has she quit menstruating?

If you answered yes to these questions, please seek help.

Treatment for Anorexia

When someone is diagnosed with anorexia, she is classed as low, intermediate, or high risk depending on how she rates on several tests.

- Low-risk people are starting to control their body and are losing weight but have not stopped menstruating or become excessively thin. They mainly need nutritional and psychological counseling.
- Intermediate-risk people are becoming visibly thin, have quit menstruating, and are acting moody and depressed. In addition to nutritional and psychological counseling, they need nutritional supplements to increase their daily intake as well as help to tolerate larger meals. One especially effective program for people of intermediate

risk is the residential treatment center. Here women live together in an environment where their meals are cooked for them, and their intake is closely monitored. They receive counseling and help from other health-care agencies like doctors, nutritionists, or hospitals as needed and benefit from seeing and talking with others who are dealing with similar issues.

• The high-risk group, those with extreme cases of anorexia, must be hospitalized and given nutrients intravenously to prevent death. Their image of themselves is usually so distorted, and their refusal to eat so ingrained, that it is difficult to reteach them to eat. It is a long, hard road back to health. On the bright side, treatment programs for anorexia are becoming more successful all the time.

BULIMIA

Betsy appears to have everything going for her. She has a full-ride scholarship to her college of choice, she belongs to a sorority, regularly attends social functions, and dates different guys. Although a normal body weight, she constantly thinks about food and her weight. No one knows that Betsy frequently starves herself, then binges, and when she has eaten too much, vomits. Betsy has bulimia.

Like anorexia, the person with bulimia constantly thinks about food and her body weight. But unlike the person with anorexia, who has an iron grip on her fork and radically limits her calorie intake, the bulimic goes on binge, eating episodes of anywhere from one-thousand to several thousands of calories at a time. Then to prevent any weight gain, she vomits or uses laxatives to purge the food from her system.

Why Do People Become Bulimic?

Like anorexia, defining the cause of bulimia is difficult. Some people begin bulimic patterns after a long series of unsuccessful diets. Obsessed with their weight, they intensely restrict calories and then find themselves starved to the point that they can't control their eating. But usually there are issues and problems from the person's past that start the bulimic cycle. Commonly, bulimics are raised in families that focus on big meals and socializing around the dinner table. Food is always involved in celebrations and hearty eating is encouraged. But when this same child is told she also must be thin, she sees her only alternative is to eat the large quantities of food and then undo any possible weight gain by fasting or vomiting. Other common characteristics among

WIDE ANGLE

Check Yourself Out

Ask yourself the following questions to better understand which of these principles you're strongest and weakest in.

Provision: I regularly recognize God's provision. I'm genuinely thankful for the food I have.

1	2	3	4	5	6	7	8	9	10

Perspective: I'm conscious of what I eat, but I wouldn't consider myself as a "stomach worshipper."

1	2	3	4	5	6	7	8	9	10

Portions: I don't eat too much, and you'll rarely find me lounging around letting the pounds pile on.

1	2	3	4	5	6	7	8	9	10

Praise: I am involved in a regular praise time. I constantly thank God for the things He's provided for me.

1	2	3	4	5	6	7	8	9	10

bulimics are a high degree of social anxiety and difficulty making friends. They often seek confirmation of their self-worth from others and feel that being thin will gain someone's favor. Depression is also high among bulimics. But other times, the person seems well adjusted, and she doesn't let her bingeing interfere with her work or social activities until serious medical complications arise. In a society that favors skinny women, bulimia is practically accepted as a way for upper-class women to deal with the frequent high-fat, high-calorie dinners and cocktail parties and still maintain their figures. But the physical effects will take their toll.

Physical Consequences

Bulimia often goes undetected because it is practiced in secret, but the symptoms after an episode are very clear. After eating such a tremendous amount of food, the person will have swollen hands and feet, bloating, fatigue, headache, nausea, and pain. As the person repeats and repeats the pattern of rigid dieting, followed by the bingeing and then the purging, she begins to face serious medical consequences.

• Fluid and electrolyte imbalance can lead to abnormal heart rhythms and injury to the kidneys.

• Vomiting causes irritation and infection to the esophagus, salivary glands, pharynx, and causes erosion of the teeth.

• Eyes can become red from the pressure of vomiting.

• Laxatives can damage the lower intestinal tract and repeated use leads to death from poisoning.

THE BOTTOM LINE

Common Factors among People with Bulimia

1. Low self-esteem. They think that if only they could be thin they would be happy.
2. Depression
3. Need to please others
4. Compulsive
5. Often children of alcoholics or abusive parents

Conquering Bulimia

Those with bulimia know the consequences of their behavior, realize it's abnormal, and feel deeply ashamed about it. They usually feel inadequate, are unable to control their eating behavior, and most are clinically depressed. The goal in helping people overcome bulimia is to help them gain control of their eating and establish regular eating patterns. Through counseling they come to understand that eating nutritious foods in the right proportions can bring them satisfaction and not make them fat. As for anorexia, treatment is a combination of psychological and nutritional counseling. Other recommendations for someone struggling with bulimia include:

• Eat snacks and meals sitting down.
• Plan meals and snacks and record food in a log before it is eaten.
• Plan meals that require the use of utensils and avoid finger food.

If you suspect someone you know has bulimia, ask yourself the following questions:

1. Does her weight fluctuate more than ten pounds up or down over a short amount of time?
2. Does she seem obsessed about her weight and food?
3. Does she make statements like, "If only I were thin. . ."?
4. Does she seem depressed?

If you answered yes to these questions, the chances are high that the person has bulimia. Help is available. Encourage that person to seek help.

WHAT YOU CAN DO

The media shouts the message that girls and women need to be thin to be beautiful and happy. Many normal-weight girls as young as ten years old are worried about their weight and are on diets. How can we counteract this lie and keep our children from developing an eating disorder? There are definite steps to take. If you are a parent or work with young children:

- Be careful not to discuss your own weight in front of children.
- Choose your words wisely when discussing your child's weight.
- Rather than classify foods as good or bad, talk about portion sizes and healthy food choices.
- Serve nutritional meals and snacks.
- Exemplify good eating and exercise habits yourself.
- Respect and value young people for who they are and teach them to respect and value themselves.

WIDE ANGLE

A Testimony

"When I was young, I competed in gymnastics. But when I hit puberty, my body changed. I gained weight and my gymnastics suffered. I thought that if I lost weight the coach would like me more, and I would be perceived as a better gymnast. So I became obsessed about my weight and didn't eat any fat, sugar, and very little carbohydrates. It wasn't until I collapsed in a floor routine that anyone confronted me about my problem. I was diagnosed with anorexia, received treatment, and fortunately today, I'm still alive."

—Name withheld, Austin, Texas

Section 8
Reengineer Your Whole Life

Forming Habits That Help

FOOD ON THE BRAIN

"Timid roach, why be so shy?
We are brothers, thou and I.
In the midnight, like thyself,
I explore the pantry shelf."
                    —Christopher Morley

Doesn't it always happen this way? You've just begun what you believe to be a smashing start to your new diet, but it seems you just can't think of anything else but food! It is as if the moment you decided to "diet," food became an obsession. Suddenly, you are transfixed by any mention of food, let alone the sight of it.

In order to create habits that are positive and productive, the old habits have to be broken—including the definition of "diet." Habits are difficult to break—just go watch the movie *Alive*.

These are **not** the best ways to avoid eating too much:
- eating on the scale
- using small plates
- eating in front of the mirror
- always eating with someone of the opposite sex
- telling yourself all the different ways you could improve each body part
- evaluating your body mass index (BMI) before every meal

THINK OF IT THIS WAY:

Would you ever go on a "diet" from God's Word? What would the results be? In the end, would you be a stronger, healthier Christian? Probably not. That is because we are to crave God's Word like a baby craves its mother's milk. . .daily!! The same is true with diet and exercise. If you stop eating what your body needs and stop moving, then you'll become unhealthy and weak.

Where do your "hard to break" habits fall?
1. You eat to:
    a. fill your body with the nutrition it needs to function at its best.
    b. satisfy your cravings.
    c. fill empty spaces of time in front of the TV because you are bored.
2. Your goal in "dieting" is:
    a. being able to go out for a deliciously fattening dinner that consists of fettuccini Alfredo and tiramisu for dessert.
    b. to become a healthier, more energetic person.
    c. to fit into a size 6 no matter what the cost.
3. Your foolproof excuse for not working out is:
    a. that a jog around the block would be murder on your knees.
    b. there is just no time in between *Friends* and *ER*.
    c. that you never seem to see any results around the hip and thigh area (even though your last attempt at a consistent workout schedule ended after a week).
    d. you've already exercised five times this week, and this is your day off.
4. Nutritional eating consists of:
    a. at least five of the daily recommended servings of fruits and vegetables.
    b. making sure you get at least one of your servings of vegetables (unfortunately, it is usually a potato in the form of chips).
    c. microwaving a frozen dinner, because cooking for one is too much trouble.
5. Your idea of a getting a good night's sleep is:
    a. being in bed before the sun comes up.
    b. getting six to eight solid hours of deep REM sleep.
    c. going to sleep with the TV on.

OUT WITH THE OLD AND IN WITH THE NEW

"Never swap horses crossing a stream."
American proverb on the idea of change.

Here is where the tough part begins. Gone are the days of naïvely believing that burgers and pizza belong to a major food group. To be successful at changing any habit, a major overhaul in your thinking needs to take place. All things worth their weight usually require hard work to attain the goal. So don't be discouraged; start trying to look at your health in a whole new way. Part of that process is defining your own personal goals. (Remember, Kate Moss and Naomi Campbell are not technically classified as goals.) Be realistic, stop comparing yourself to others, and do what works for you! Diet and exercise take patience and commitment. So don't beat yourself up. Just remember. . .everything in moderation.

Seeing Is Believing
Go out to the local drugstore and plunk down a few bucks for a notebook. Start keeping a food journal—seeing it on paper will make all the difference. It's guaranteed that you'll discover what and how much food really goes into your mouth. It will open your eyes to where the changes need to be made.

Start at the Bunny Hill
Once you've noticed where you want to make changes, make sure you start small. If you change everything all at once then you will be overwhelmed and quit. Instead of taking everything you like out of your diet, start with something like how often you're allowed dinner out in a week. All the little changes will end up making all the difference in the long run. It also won't feel so drastic and you're more likely to stick with it.
   Small steps to making a big difference:
- Start drinking plenty of water—recommended daily intake is eight eight-ounce glasses. Don't worry; you won't float away.
- Instead of cold pizza for breakfast, try integrating fresh fruit into your day. Fruit is jammed with nutrients and is very low in calories. It will fill you up fast and has no drawbacks to it at all—so eat as much as you want in the morning.
- Become a forager. Eat small, healthy meals throughout your whole day. It may seem like you are eating all day, but it will ward off hunger attacks (basically, that candy bar won't be calling your name as loudly come three o'clock in the afternoon).
- Start moving—any way you can. Just start walking around the neighborhood.
- Quit snacking in front of the TV. You won't realize how much you are eating and those calories will be wasted.
- Try to think of food in terms of the nutrition value it will bring to you. It will then have a real purpose and won't be a negative thing.
- Worry more about what you are eating and not as much about how much.

- Stop reading beauty magazines. Instead of encouraging you, they will take your focus off what really matters. . .your health and fitness level.
- Above all, remember that your body is the temple of the Holy Spirit and as such you need to take care of it the best you can.

(Remember, just modify a few habits. Don't go climbin' every mountain just yet.)

EXERCISE? IT'S NOT ALL TORTURE

Exercise doesn't always have to be a painful thing (just sometimes). Not everyone enjoys jogging. Get creative. You will be more likely to stick with something if you love it. It's just like a hobby you like; i.e., photography—it's fun, creative, and exciting. Well, exercise can be too. It's all in the way you look at it.

Looking for exercise in all the wrong places? Here are some ideas:

Taking advantage of the different seasons is a great way to add variety, and depending on where you are, there are many ways to get out and enjoy the scenery. There are a million (or close to) different things you can do.

Summer—obviously the weather is conducive to being outdoors, so get out of the AC and sweat a little. **Fall** is also a beautiful time to be outdoors.

Try. . .

- Rollerblading. If speed and being daring are what you are looking for, then this is for you. (Just be sure to wear knee and elbow pads.)
- Swimming. Do some laps in the local community pool. It can be relaxing and is a great cardiovascular workout.
- Hiking and biking. Do some research on where there are trails and paths. It's doubly great; you can enjoy nature and raise your metabolism.
- Canoeing, kayaking, rowing—fun ways to enjoy the water.
- Riding. Sometimes local stables offer a flat rate for an hour or two of riding.

Winter and **spring** are more difficult to be outside, but it is still doable. You can choose to do more indoors too. Try. . .

- Dancing. It's indoors and is a fun way to get a great cardiovascular workout. There are many types of dancing, i.e., swing, line, ballroom. You do need a partner for these, so this could be a deterrent.

- Skiing. Harder to do in flat environments, but remember there is always cross-county skiing too.
- Ice skating. Takes some coordination, but it is fun.
- Videos. Different workout videos are a great way to stay in from the outdoors and still get a good workout.
- Cleaning the house. As fun as this isn't, it does get you moving. All that scrubbing is a good way to burn some calories.

SET MINI-GOALS

Your mini-goals should be succeeding in those small adjustments that you make. These will turn into longer-term goals as you progress. Don't start with taking off twenty pounds in a month. Start with five pounds and go from there. Same thing with exercise. Start walking three times a week and build up to four or five times. From there perhaps you can find a jogging track and alternate walking and jogging. Just build up. As you get better maybe you'll find a 5K run you can attempt.

AQUA

Don't underestimate the power of water. Our bodies consist of about 65 percent water and it is essential in all of our bodily functions—including brain function. So put down the soda, coffee, and even juice, and get your eight glasses of H_2O per day. You won't believe the difference it will make.

PLANNING?

As stressful and time-consuming as you think it may be, planning actually saves time and takes the pressure off of you during your daily routine. Make a chart at the beginning of the week to plan your meals. Planning your workouts is also a good idea. Seeing it down on paper will help solidify it in your mind and you will

Use Your Head

wow!

"If a man empties his purse into his head, no man can take it away from him. An investment in knowledge always pays the best interest."
—Benjamin Franklin

be more likely to actually get out of the house instead of parking yourself in front of the TV. You can avoid some of those bad habits by doing a little planning beforehand.

IDEAS FOR YOUR PLAN

Get Spiritual

The best support you will ever find is from God. As a believer, you are equipped with the best advice and direction possible. . .Scripture. God's Word *is* sufficient for all things. So get into the Word!! Be sure to keep your priorities in check. Your relationship with Christ should be your number one goal. If you are focused solely on your body and the way it looks, then that will detract from your focus on God. Besides, God is far more concerned with the condition of your heart and how it looks rather than the how svelte your body is. So be wise.

Ask yourself questions to see where you're really at. These are questions only you can answer. So be honest and then reevaluate.
- How often are you in God's Word?
- In who or what do you find your identity?
- Are you spending more time worrying about how you look on the outside or how God sees you on the inside?
- Who are you trying to please?

EDUCATION

Believe it or not, part of finding support is gathering a base of information for you. The more you know, the easier it will be to evaluate what works best for you. Even Oprah has some good ideas (too bad Rosie, the cook, isn't one of them).

Here are some ideas of people and places where you can find supportive and helpful information:
- Ask your doctor. He/she will be a wealth of information about good, basic nutrition.
- See a nutritionist. Set up an appointment for an evaluation.

wow!

Stay Away

Top people not to ask help from when you are trying to lose weight:
1. David Letterman—does he really know his cuts of meat?
2. Your best friend—who can eat whatever she wants and still look great.
3. Your mother—who cooks everything with butter.
4. John the Baptist—"No locusts, no honey."

It isn't that expensive for a one-time visit. They can give you creative ways to cook nutritiously.

- When you join a local gym, they often provide trainers or weight loss and fitness classes on the premises. Take advantage. Get evaluated. Ask questions. They will help you get started or help you increase your fitness level.

- Go to the local library. There are hundreds of different cookbooks, magazines and videos on health, nutrition, and exercise. Even magazines, such as *Good Housekeeping*, *Self*, and *Prevention* have good ideas. These resources can provide new ways to spice up your workout or give helpful low-fat recipes.

- Get on the Internet. There is more information than you will know what to do with. Many sites also provide links to other helpful places you can find information. Some helpful sites are:
  http://www.bobgreenonline.com
  http://www.onhealth.com
  http://www.eatright.org (American Dietetic Association)
  http://www.prevention.com
  http://www.self.com

Join a support group, or start your own! The more the merrier.
There are a variety of groups to help give you ideas and motivate you. For instance, if you absolutely love running, find the local running fanatics and work out with them. Those people will also be a good source of information for you. Not only that, but it will be an inspiration for you to be around people who like the same thing.

If you aren't sure what is available in your local area, just start a support group of your own. Get a group of friends together and start throwing around ideas, sharing your struggles, and giving each other encouragement. Two heads are always better than one. Plus, it isn't nearly as much fun alone.

Dieting with Another Person

FIND A PARTNER IN CRIME

Find somebody you trust, because this is a fabulous way to get support and encouragement. It is also far less lonely to have someone going through the same thing you are. So find someone that you can laugh with, cry with, and confide in.

A partner should be a great friend who knows just what you are going through. Don't pick someone who would say:

- "Get your behind in gear. I know where you live."
- "How much did you lose last week?"
- "You're going to eat t*hat*?"
- "Doesn't the Bible talk about being a glutton?"
- "You're never going to catch a guy."
- "What size are those?"
- "How many fat grams are in *that*?"
- "What's your problem? It's all about willpower."
- "Did you say you wanted to be married?"

Would you be a good partner?

1. Are you sensitive to others' dilemmas?

1	2	3	4	5	6	7	8	9	10
Sometimes, but only when interested					Could care less			Generally feel others' pain	

2. Are you available when someone really needs you?

1	2	3	4	5	6	7	8	9	10
Not a chance				Only if it is convenient					24 hours, 7 days a week

3. Are you faithful to pray for others?

1	2	3	4	5	6	7	8	9	10

Pray? What does   Only when it comes   Rug burns on

that mean?   to mind   the knees

4. Can you laugh at yourself?

1	2	3	4	5	6	7	8	9	10

I never laugh   If it is about   I laugh at

                   someone else   everything

5. Are you willing to be accountable?

1	2	3	4	5	6	7	8	9	10

"Mums" the word   Yeah, but only so far   Let the wind

                                             blow in

Results

5–15: What kind of a friend are you anyway? It would be best to start with your attitude.

16–35: You still need to work on some things, but having a partner will be a good learning experience for you.

36–50: You must be Dear Abby or something. You're a great friend.

ACCOUNTABILITY

If you know that your partner will be asking you if you would like to fork over your food journal, you may be less likely to reach for that next piece of cake. This will keep you on track and honest.

PRAY TOGETHER

This is the best way to encourage each other. Pray for each other's struggles and give praise for the needs God has answered. When you see a habit that needs to be changed, lift it up in prayer—together.

Cook Together

Find recipes you both like and try them out. This way you can experiment without having a ton of food left over that you may not eat.

Work Out Together

Working out with someone is much more fun. You can laugh (or cry) when you fall on your rollerblades, you can push each other to go farther than you thought you could, and you can be far more adventurous. So get out there and try some new sports. It is more motivating to be with a friend than all on your own.

One Day at a Time

Remember, start with changing small things about how you eat. Remembering what nutritional value a candy bar has may deter your willingness to eat it. Nothing happens overnight and this certainly won't either. Unfortunately, you will fail at times. But don't get discouraged and give up. The best of people take a fall. But what makes them the "best" is that they get up, learn from their mistakes, and move on.

WOW!

Making Healthy Eating a Lasting Habit, Not a Passing Phase.

"It wasn't until I reached my early twenties that I finally got a clue about what health and fitness were all about. I wasn't terribly overweight, but my sisters used to tell me that I needed to lose weight or I would never 'catch a guy.' For some reason I never listened to them. I watched as they had their own weight fluctuations up and down the scale. They would take herbal pills and fast to lose weight. In the meantime, I didn't worry a ton about what I ate. I just tried to keep my focus on the right things. Now at twenty-seven, I am satisfied with how I look and I don't struggle with where my weight is or isn't—guy or no guy."
—Sheryl, London, England

- Be aware of your mood when you don't feel like working out, so next time you can find ways to motivate yourself out of the house.
- Be conscious of what is entering your mouth. Look at your food in terms of what nutritional value it holds.
- Make sure that your emotions aren't what leads you to eat. This is a huge stumbling block for many people. Our culture eats when it is sad, depressed, happy, and when celebrating. Find other things to focus on during those times. Make yourself busy. The result will be

that you won't correlate those emotions with food.

- Eat a variety of different things. That way you won't get tired of just having the same thing. Cook with fresh herbs and spices. That gives food great taste.

Actions. . .

"Thought is the blossom; language the bud; action the fruit behind it."

DON'T FORGET —Ralph Waldo Emerson

- Be smart about all that is "low fat" or "fat free." Just because they are called Nestle Sweet Escapes and they are low fat, doesn't mean you can eat the whole bag. You may just end up "escaping" a little too much. If you are going to have sweets, don't waste the calories. Have something really yummy.

- Don't stress out. Technically, nothing is off-limits. It is all about balance. Don't tell yourself you can't have that chocolate cake. You'll just want it even more. Eat a piece (but not the whole thing), and make sure you have eaten a healthy, balanced diet beforehand.

To Infinity and Beyond

The way to look at the dieting process is to see it as a journey. As each day passes, you will notice that all of the small changes you made are making a big difference. Just remember; it isn't going to happen overnight. But, finally, after hard work, sweat, and tears, the results you envisioned for the future will be here; but it takes commitment and endurance.

Your attitude will make all the difference. Don't be pessimistic. It won't take you very far. You'll end up quitting. Be hopeful about the future. You are making changes that will improve your quality of life (and you don't want to end up aging before your time, do you?).

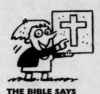

Get Ready

"Therefore gird up the loins of your mind, be sober, and rest your hope fully upon the grace that is to be brought to you at the revelation of Jesus Christ" (I Peter 1:13 NKJV).

THE BIBLE SAYS

THE FLAG OF CONSCIOUSNESS

Imagine for a moment. You're standing around a flagpole with your family. Flag in hand, you attach it to the rope. You hold hands as the flag is raised. Together, you repeat "Better Eating" over and over. The flag reaches the top. You raise your hands. In this moment you feel an incredible sense of family unity. Actually, you've never felt so close to them. You even begin to tear up thinking that you're all about to enter your diets as a team. What an awesome moment.

Then you realize the most embarrassing thing. You're sitting up in bed with your hands above your head. Your spouse is staring at you with one of those scared "deer in the headlights" looks. It was all a dream.

It can be tough, but joining together as a family and working together to improve the quality of your meals and your health can be more than a dream. It's also necessary that you do this together. Doing this alone, or apart from each other, can work, but there won't be the sense of camaraderie. And camaraderie is part of what we're going for here.

GOOD FAMILY EATING

You might read that above title and think, *OK, great idea, people. But, in MY family, there's a lot of work to be done. And we don't even eat meals together. So, how in the world can we begin eating well?*

It can be stressful, but it can also be very wonderful. Consider some of the following ideas to get your family on track:

Eat together
Simple as it might sound, eating together is probably your biggest hurdle. And, if your schedule is like many others, clearing this jump will take a monumental family resolution.

Eating together is more about togetherness than it is about good eating. Sure, we're asking you to eat together to begin forming some proper familywide (no pun intended) eating habits. But eating together as a family gives you time to talk about your day. It gives you time to grow together. Eating together won't just afford you time to strive toward health; it will give you an opportunity to grow together, share experiences, and form a bond.

An Eating Plan

This book contains a lot of information about health and dieting. And, you've probably found ideas stuffed in these pages that give you direction for what you'd like to implement in your family.

Whatever dieting plan you feel comfortable adopting, adapt it to fit your family and go for it. Once you've established your plan, have family members sign a covenant to keep their diet and exercise plan. Then, ask the following questions:

- Is it realistic? Does this eating plan offer enough nourishment for my family?
- Is it thought out? Is this eating plan really a healthier alternative to what we already have?
- Is it specific? Are meals specifically described and designated for certain days?

Say "NO!" to Junk

If you're a typical family, there's a disease in your house. It's called junk food. Yep, it's probably lurking in the corners of your cabinets. And if you've talked about a family diet plan before, there's probably some hidden in your kids' rooms or your spouse's secret hiding place.

One sure way to keep your family away from junk food is to get rid of it, and don't bring any into your home. This way, you can easily monitor the amount of junk food they eat. . .because there won't be any! Instead, keep a supply of healthy snacks on hand: carrots, celery, rice cakes, crackers, cold water, juice, etc.

"What I Ate" Chart

Help your family be more conscious of what they eat by creating a "What I Ate" chart and hanging it on the refrigerator. At the evening meal, pass the chart around and have family members write in what they ate for each meal. Then, sometime after the meal (maybe during a family walk!?), ask all of them to evaluate how they ate that day. Then, ask them how they might eat better the following day.

	Family Member 1	Family Member 2	Family Member 3	Family Member 4
Breakfast				
Lunch				
Dinner				

Not After Six

The people who create commercials aren't stupid. Ever watch television after dinnertime? If you do, you'll notice a lot of advertising for fast-food restaurants, snack foods, and desserts. Advertisers know what they're doing. They know that we get hungry at night. (Consider that, after dinner, you'll go another thirteen hours before you eat again).

This rule will be tough. Establish a "no eating after dinner" rule. That means after dinner, the kitchen is closed. If your family totally revolts and offers to trade you for a large pizza or chocolate cake, offer to have healthy snack food available after dinner. If you do this, put it in a place where others won't be tempted to eat other types of food.

Good Morning!

Someone once said, "Eat like a king at breakfast, a prince at lunch, and a pauper at dinner." That's not just a catchy phrase; it's also good advice. How do you make that happen in your family? Consider serving good-sized family breakfasts.

Eat healthy at breakfast. Most cereal has a lot of junk in it. And, eating mostly sugar in the morning will leave children hungry later. Give them fruit, oatmeal, toast, and other substantive things.

THE FLIP SIDE

Family exercise. It might feel as impressive a task as getting a full-time job licking stamps at the post office. Most experts will tell you that dieting without exercise doesn't work. Exercise is important. Use some of these ideas to help your family grasp the essential other side of good eating—good exercise.

AFTER-DINNER WALKS

We've already suggested having dinner together. After an evening meal, consider going on a family walk. It's a great time to get to know your neighbors, discover new things in your neighborhood, and get healthy at the same time.

FUN EXERCISE

When you begin thinking about family exercise, things that were fun in the recent past become tools for fun exercise. Consider going bowling, roller (or even in-line) skating, sledding, or swimming together.

It's also OK to ask each family member to be involved in some sort of formal exercise throughout the week. And you can encourage family members to find a way to make their exercise fun. Consider having family competitions for some of the exercises your family is involved in.

NO TELEVISION

One of the biggest deterrents to family or individual exercise is the television. Sometimes, it's easier to get involved in watching people work out than it is actually working out. You CAN beat the TV! How? Establish rules for when it can be on. Consider having family members vote on what shows and times are OK to watch. Then, establish yourself as the rule enforcer.

SOMETHING DIFFICULT

Technology is great. Modern conveniences are wonderful. And, while those things have advanced society, they've also made us dependent on them. How can you embrace technological advances, but also use them to establish family exercise?

Simple. Do something the hard way. Consider using a very old (push type—not motorized) lawn mower. Use a rake instead of a leaf blower. Wash your clothes in a bathtub. Walk to the store instead of driving. Park in the back of the parking lot of your grocery store and walk to the entrance (you'll not only save a closer spot for an older person, you'll get in shape!).

Simply step back from your everyday life and look at what you use to make your life easier, then get rid of that for a whole week. You'll be amazed at what you accomplish.

PERSPECTIVE

Getting focused on your family diet doesn't always mean talking about or doing things that relate specifically to your diet. Since you and every member is a wonderful awesome creation of God, try gathering at the end of every day and giving Him the glory for creating you, for providing for you, and for giving you the strength to make it in life, and even in your diets. Guide yourself in this process by reading Psalm 136 together every evening before you go to bed. Have one person read the first part of each verse, then have the family read responsively, "His love endures forever" or however it's listed in your Bible.

THE HEART OF IT ALL

Stop for a moment, close your eyes, and imagine that you're God. Now imagine that you're looking at your family. What might He say about your diet? What might He say about your exercise? What might God say about the health of your family? Write some ideas below.

_____

_____

_____

_____

_____

_____

_____

God wants us to be healthy, but He doesn't provide us with an easy three-step plan for getting healthy. That's because your family, like all families, is a unique and special creation. Establishing a family health objective, trying family exercises, and even trying to change the diet of your family isn't easy.

The Parental Pass

It's your kids' graduation day. You've waited for this event your entire life. They've crammed a four-year degree into six years, their tuition left you with about $1.98 in your savings account, and you're convinced you've funded several out-of-the-country business trips for the execs at your long-distance service. Pride fills you as your children confidently walk across the stage, grab the diploma, shake a few hands, and head off. And then it happens. Your student passes the microphone, stops, wavers for a moment, then begins to speak. You're squinting your eyes and hoping he doesn't utter something rude or embarrassing.

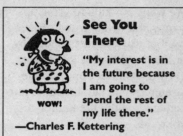

See You There

"My interest is in the future because I am going to spend the rest of my life there."

—Charles F. Kettering

wow!

"I'd just like to thank my parents for teaching me to eat right. Their influence on my nutrition has made me the person I am today."

Yeah, right. Okay, maybe it's a bit far-fetched to think that the one thought on your child's mind on her graduation day will be how you taught her to eat, but consider that how she eats makes her part of who she is. While what you teach her about food probably won't be on the front of her mind, it will influence how she acts and what she accomplishes.

Helping your child graduate into life with healthy eating habits might feel a bit daunting. Consider the following strategies for passing on healthy eating habits to him or her.

Life 101

We want our kids to grow up happy and healthy. But growing up that way doesn't happen by accident. It takes a lot of work. Let's chat about some simple strategies you can implement to cement healthy life habits in your kids.

SMALLER EYES

A plate is a big thing. And some plates take a lot to fill up. So, when you sit down for meals, it's easy to put a lot of food on your plate.

Help your kids understand the value of eating slow. Try something like having everyone eat a bite together and not take another one until you instruct.

WIDE ANGLE

Habits

Before you begin trying to change the eating habits of your family, it's best to consider how your family might feel about this idea. In the space below, write out how you think your family might feel about what you might suggest. Once you've written down your thoughts, read back over them and consider if your family is ready to have their eating habits improved.

_____

_____

_____

_____

And encourage your family to take smaller portions. One surefire way to do this is prepare their plates and *then* take the plates to the table. Tell them that they can always have more, but only if they're still hungry.

But you might have another idea for helping your kids take smaller portions, or eat less. If you do, write them here.

_____

_____

_____

_____

PATIENCE PAYS OFF

It's three o'clock in the afternoon. You see your child exit the pantry with a bag of chips. What should you do?

a. Drop some ants in the bag while he's not looking?
b. Complain that he doesn't eat healthier?
c. Help him understand how patience pays off?

Okay, we set you up. The correct answer is "C" (but doesn't "A" sound a little fun?).

How does having patience pay off and help your kid establish a healthy habit for his life? Simple. If you'll teach your kid that *waiting* for his favorite snack is better than giving in and eating it when the urge hits, you'll help him understand the value that food has. Most snack food is eaten when the urge hits, not when someone is hungry. Tell your children this, and help them evaluate whether they're really hungry, or if they're just craving a taste.

Getting your kids to wait until they're hungry to eat isn't easy. Try:

- Having them go do something else for ten minutes. If they're still hungry after that, reconsider your alternatives.
- Giving them a healthy alternative to what they want.
- If you feel that they're not really hungry, hold fast to your standard. It might be difficult, but your child will learn that family health is important.

What other "waiting" ideas do you have?

_____

_____

_____

_____

_____

_____

FOUR BIGGIES

What are the four biggies? Simply put, these are four things to consider before putting any food into your mouth. These four biggies are built on the idea that *everything* you put into your body affects you. Read through them and consider how you might help your children understand these.

My Brain:

Some foods can alter how your brain works. Caffeine, for instance, gives some people that extra jolt they need in the afternoon. Sugar causes smaller children to become hyperactive. The substances that are brought together to create certain foods can alter brain activity. They change your ability to focus, have patience—and in extreme instances, can cause other problems, including an inability to sleep at night or focus for longer periods of time.

The first biggie to teach your children is that some foods affect your brain. So, teach them to ask this question before they eat any food.

• What effect will this food have on my mind?

My Bones:

OK, it's true that not many foods actually harm your bones, but some foods actually help your bones. Milk, for instance, provides calcium. And, remember that your teeth are bones. So, things like candy, sugared drinks, sticky foods, and the like can do more harm than good. While your kids might not think it's a whole lot of fun to have a glass of milk instead of a huge can of soda, standing by this consideration will help them grow stronger, and they'll avoid LARGE dentist bills later in life. What one rule can you pass on to your kids in this area? Teach them to ask:

• How will this food affect my teeth and bones?

My Tissue:

This category is both an inside and outside focus. And it's one that your kid might not consider.

Certain foods affect the interior of your body. Too much roughage can overwork your body. Too much meat can be bad for your body. And, oftentimes, some foods have an effect on your skin. Onions (for example) can make some people's skin (and breath!) stink. Hot peppers make other people's scalps sweat. It's important for your kids to consider that whatever they put into their bodies affects the interior of it.

Teach your kids to ask this important question about what they put into their bodies:

- What will this food do to the way I smell? How will this food affect my insides?

My Chemicals:

What are you allergic to? What is your child allergic to? God made each of us unique. Different personalities. Different likes and dislikes. And, a different tolerance for foods. Strawberries make some people break out. Some spices can cause people to have an allergic reaction. This question isn't one your kids are likely to stop and consider a lot, especially if they've never had any difficulties. But if your child is prone to allergic reactions or severe upset stomachs as a result of some foods, this question is one of vital importance. Teach him to ask:

- Am I allergic to this food? What effect will this food have on me?

GARBAGE COLLECTING

Whatever your child puts into their minds will come out their mouths. The same holds true for their bodies. If they fill it with junk, they'll not live up to the dreams God has for them. If, however, they fill themselves with good food, the chances are better that they'll have the strength and energy to reach whatever goal they strive for. It's the old "Garbage In—Garbage Out" rule. And it's totally true. So, ultimately, you want to teach your child to ask:

- What will this food produce in my life? How will it help me accomplish what God has for me to do?

PASSING ON THE RULES

You've heard the old song, "It only takes a spark to get a fire going"? Right? Well, the same holds true with helping your children live with healthy eating habits when they leave your nest. You're the spark. The way you live feeds the fire.

Whatever your strategy for helping your children live with healthy eating habits, there are four simple guidelines that we'd like you to remember as you forge ahead with helping them live out what you've taught them about eating.

Preach the Habit

Your kids probably hear you spewing out rules all the time. And, you might begin to wonder how much of that gets stuck in their brains and how much of it they just forget. Truth is, your kids secretly depend on you to set the standard for them. They're waiting for you to give them boundaries. Even though they might verbally reject the ideas you set before them, chances are they'll adopt them sooner or later. And, if you're convinced that your children ignore *everything* you have to say, you might want to consider strategically placing someone in your family that they *will* listen to. Invite someone over for dinner who eats very healthily, and have her discuss her eating habits (just make sure this doesn't come off scripted. . .your kids *will* notice).

Do whatever you can to give them guidelines for healthy eating. You can even use the guidelines in this book (feel free to copy everything in this book into your life).

Live the Habit

There's an old story about a clown who noticed that the circus he'd worked for his entire life had caught fire. The big top was going up in flames, and innocent circusgoers were trapped. Thinking fast, the clown grabbed the first thing he could find (a unicycle) and, in costume, went to town to see if he could gather people to help extinguish the fire. The clown rode up and down the streets of the small town yelling and screaming for help. But, with each home he passed, he was met with laughter. It seemed the people of the town couldn't take a clown seriously. The circus burned to the ground; many lives were lost. *(Story from* Hot Illustrations for Youth Talks, *volume 1, pages 68–69.)*

If we attempt to tell our kids how to change their eating habits, but refuse to change our own, we'll look like a clown screaming for help. What we're saying won't take, and our kids will ignore us. So, preach all you want about healthy eating to your children. But follow that up with changing your life. How to do that is very simple. Just do everything you're asking your kids to do. Change the mood of your family from whatever it is now to total family health. Then, lead the way by being the first person to exercise, the first to eat healthy, and the first to change your life.

Public Reinforcement

OK, so you've got all of that stuff down. And you're ready to take what you've been teaching your family on the road. You're ready for whatever the fast-food or upscale restaurant dishes out. How can you encourage your kids to eat healthy when they're out?

Consistency is key here. Help them learn how to eat on their own by giving them parameters when they're at restaurants with you. This might require some research into what types of food these places offer, but your work will pay off. Once you've researched some caloric, fat, and protein contents, create some general guidelines for your kids. Reinforce this by taking them out regularly (they'll love this, until they catch on to what you're up to) and showing them how they can eat healthily. If you'll do this, and remain consistent, they'll catch on, and it'll become part of who they are.

Private Encouragement

Above everything we've talked about in this chapter, remember this: Your children will learn from you. They're watching what you eat. They're paying attention to your exercise schedule. And, most likely, they'll model what you live.

Encourage your kids to eat right, exercise, and be aware of how they're treating their bodies. Do this by eating right yourself. Exercise, if not for yourself, so

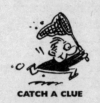

Here's an Idea

CATCH A CLUE

Want to help your family eat less? Buy smaller plates. And get rid of your old ones so you're not tempted to bring them out when you're really hungry or when the others are dirty.

they'll catch on to the necessity of personal health. And, above all, reinforce everything good you're modeling by directing them to God. Tell them that God made them. And, it's important to take care of what God created.

NOTES

NOTES

Inspirational Library

Beautiful purse/pocket-size editions of Christian classics bound in flexible leatherette. These books make thoughtful gifts for everyone on your list, including yourself!

When I'm on My Knees   The highly popular collection of devotional thoughts on prayer, especially for women.
      Flexible Leatherette. $4.97

The Bible Promise Book   Over 1,000 promises from God's Word arranged by topic. What does God promise about matters like: Anger, Illness, Jealousy, Love, Money, Old Age, and Mercy? Find out in this book!
      Flexible Leatherette. $3.97

Daily Wisdom for Women   A daily devotional for women seeking biblical wisdom to apply to their lives. Scripture taken from the New American Standard Version of the Bible.
      Flexible Leatherette. $4.97

My Daily Prayer Journal   Each page is dated and features a Scripture verse and ample room for you to record your thoughts, prayers, and praises. One page for each day of the year.
      Flexible Leatherette. $4.97

Available wherever books are sold.
Or order from:

Barbour Publishing, Inc.
P.O. Box 719
Uhrichsville, OH 44683
www.barbourbooks.com

If you order by mail, add $2.00 to your order for shipping.
Prices are subject to change without notice.